How Do You Feel?

How Do You Feel?

One Doctor's Search for
Humanity in Medicine

Jessi Gold, MD, MS

Simon Element

New York   London   Toronto   Sydney   New Delhi

SIMON ELEMENT

An Imprint of Simon & Schuster, LLC
1230 Avenue of the Americas
New York, NY 10020

First Simon Element hardcover edition October 2024

SIMON ELEMENT is a trademark of Simon & Schuster, LLC

Simon & Schuster: Celebrating 100 Years of Publishing in 2024

For information about special discounts for bulk purchases, please contact Simon & Schuster Special Sales at 1-866-506-1949 or business@simonandschuster.com.

The Simon & Schuster Speakers Bureau can bring authors to your live event. For more information or to book an event, contact the Simon & Schuster Speakers Bureau at 1-866-248-3049 or visit our website at www.simonspeakers.com.

Interior design by Davina Mock-Maniscalco

Manufactured in the United States of America

1   3   5   7   9   10   8   6   4   2

Library of Congress Cataloging-in-Publication Data has been applied for.

ISBN 978-1-9821-9977-7
ISBN 978-1-9821-9979-1 (ebook)

I'm not a victim or a survivor. I'm not brave or strong.
I'm just a little human with a lot more being.

—Kiana Azizian

For the humans and the ones who lift them up,
and perhaps most specifically, the ones in healthcare who are both

Author's Note

IT'S IMPORTANT FOR anyone reading this book to know that the patients you will read about in these pages are composites, meaning that I used details from a number of people and sources so as to protect any one individual's identity. They are inspired not just by the healthcare workers whom I treat in my clinic—many of whom have read the text and agreed to having some of their story included—but also the friends, family, and colleagues across the country who work as doctors, nurses, physician associates, therapists, and in other medical professions. I've also incorporated details I gleaned from my interviews with more than forty healthcare workers over the course of writing this book. My therapist, however, despite the pseudonym, is entirely real.

The stories described here take place during a time period I refer to as "the pandemic," but the book really focuses on the beginning months of March to November 2020. To tell these stories within that shortened time frame, I condensed some timelines for the patient narratives (including my own).

It's also important for readers to know that some of the information that appears in these pages might be triggering, especially for healthcare workers or anyone who lives with or loves them. If you need to take a break to grab a drink of water, or even to call your therapist, I approve! I've had to take breaks of my own at different times while in the midst of writing these stories, so I get it.

You'll find humor and a healthy sprinkling of pop culture references throughout the book. I do this not to minimize what healthcare workers go through, or what I did, but to break up the conversation a bit and lighten the mood. It's okay to laugh, and in fact I hope you do.

Finally, I write from the perspective of who I am: a white, elder-millennial woman. I try to learn as much as I can from friends and patients with different backgrounds, but I cannot speak to all the issues of well-being and identity that are interconnected within healthcare. For those topics, please look to other writers who discuss those experiences in more depth.

In my lectures, I first give my disclosures, then always start with the same slide—one meant to ask people (and myself) a question. One that allows us all to pause and reflect, something I (and most others) rarely do. Similarly, I hope you'll take the time to answer that question now, as well as at other points throughout the book.

So: *How do you feel?*

Contents

Introduction

EVERYTHING WAS FINE, until it wasn't. At least that's what I kept telling myself during the weeks, then the months, of pushing through and pushing down and flat out ignoring. *It's fine. I'm fine.* I can still do my job as a psychiatrist. I haven't made a mistake. People *need* me.

Except one day, something changed. Call it reaching a breaking point, or hitting rock bottom, but something happened that made me realize I *wasn't* fine and that I hadn't been fine for a long time.

I had trouble getting myself out of bed that morning, and after my shower, I barely managed to find a T-shirt and a clean pair of sweatpants to put on. I'm lucky that with the Zoom screen, I could get away with throwing on my work-issued fleece, which had the words "Department of Psychiatry" and my hospital's logo on it. I hoped it made me look semi-professional, but I was also completely aware that staying in pajamas all day is probably not a *great* sign. If I were my own patient, I'd be concerned.

At the computer, I remember glancing at my schedule and already feeling overwhelmed. It wasn't just the more than thirty patients I had scheduled that week; it was also the three lectures I said I would give across the hospital system and the article I had agreed to write for a magazine. *Stop, you're fine,* I told myself. I had been telling myself that a lot lately. Then, without another thought, I slipped into doctor mode and clicked open my first patient visit of the day.

On the computer screen was a sandy-haired college student

named James, who looked younger than the age listed in his medical record. After saying hi and getting a hi in return, I noted that James was scheduled for an hour rather than the thirty minutes allotted for patients who have seen me before. So, I launched into my usual new-patient spiel, since I didn't recognize his name or face. I often see ten or more patients a day, including one or two new patients. Because of that, I rarely have time to look deeply into the chart of my next patient for specifics on their psychiatric history or the reason they've made an appointment with me. Typically, during the day, I'm running on semi-autopilot: next patient, one hour, *go!* I glance at their name, open a new note, and start talking.

"It's so nice to meet you!" I said. "I'm Dr. Gold. What brings you to see me today?"

I paused and waited for James to answer, but then the pause stretched out longer, and longer still. I watched as his expression changed from apathetic to angry, and suddenly I snapped to attention. I began to wonder if maybe James didn't feel comfortable talking to me, or even being here, which wouldn't be a new experience for me as a psychiatrist. Still, I waited, refraining from saying anything. I didn't want to make assumptions when I was meeting someone for the first time.

Finally, James shifted uncomfortably and replied, "Ummm . . . I *know* you, Dr. Gold. We met three weeks ago."

I felt my stomach drop. *SHIT. SHIT. SHIT.* I tried but failed to fight my feelings of embarrassment and anxiety, or to keep my deep discomfort from showing. It's a lot harder to maintain a poker face when you're emotionally overwhelmed and exhausted. And I was more tired than I'd ever been before.

I remember immediately dressing myself down internally. *I'm horrible. I can't believe I could do that to someone. He hates me and I don't blame him because I hate me, too.* Even on the best of days, my negative self-talk can come out loud and clear.

Besides being angry at myself, I felt for my patient. My empathy was on overdrive, my mind imagining what it must feel like to be forgotten by a doctor who, only weeks earlier, had asked you to reveal your deepest, darkest secrets. I'm terrified that in one thoughtless, mistaken sentence, I had just ruptured our nascent therapeutic relationship. *Who would blame him for not wanting to see me again?*

I don't know exactly how long it was before I attempted to speak, but it felt like forever, words not coming out, stomach churning, worries swirling in my head. *I'm supposed to be here to help him. I'm supposed to have my shit together. Doctors don't make mistakes like this.*

Eventually, I took a deep breath and began speaking, nervously, "I'm *so* sorry. I don't know what to say except that I'm completely embarrassed. Since you were scheduled for an hour-long appointment, and new patients get an hour, I assumed you were new." Pinning my mistake on scheduling and logistics, I hoped that would make me look less scattered. But the voice in my head kept saying, *Nice try. He'll never buy it.*

James's face remained unflinching, but his body looked even more rigid than before. I remember that he moved his chair back from the computer screen, which suggested that he felt much more guarded than when the camera first turned on. Meanwhile, I rambled on about logistics, and I even started blaming telehealth, my *mea culpas* punctuated with apologies.

"It's fine, Dr. Gold," he finally replied. But it wasn't.

I've seen hundreds of patients in the nearly ten years since I've been practicing psychiatry after I completed medical school, and I have never, *ever* forgotten one. Yes, sometimes the details of a person's story get fuzzy (that's what notes are for), but until this moment with James I wouldn't have been able to fathom not remembering a patient I'd already met. If anything, I usually care too much about my patients, meaning I think about them after their sessions, in the evenings or on weekends, and even in my own therapist's office.

I felt like crying, which I often do when I'm anxious or mad. I didn't cry, though. This wasn't my own therapy session, after all.

We continued our conversation for a while, but it was as if I were watching myself from above, as I played the role of psychiatrist, asking questions, even throwing in a joke here or there to elicit a smile. But it was obvious that James was keeping me at an emotional distance. He responded to my questions mostly with nods and headshakes, terse yeses and nos. There was plenty of silence in between the responses, during which time my faux pas played on a continual loop, as if I could rewind to the beginning but alter the outcome. Meanwhile, outside my head, I tried to project the most charming, empathetic, attentive version of myself possible.

I began to worry that James would see through my efforts or think I was being over the top, but suddenly—and I recall this vividly now—his body relaxed and as we said goodbye, he smiled; it was a real smile. For a moment, I believed he might forgive me and be able to trust me again. Not that I could forgive myself.

1

MY FIRST DAY of pulmonology workshop in med school is impossible to forget. The professor walked in and, looking around, said what every professor seemed to say in every new class: "We'll be starting things off with an icebreaker!" That means they would inevitably continue with some version of, "As we go around the room, say your name and what specialty you want to go into." I'd been through what felt like countless iterations of this routine already.

No one said a word, but I knew we were all reacting internally with *ughs* and *not agains*. If you looked fast enough, you might even have caught some of us rolling our eyes, not just because of the monotony of the question but also because we'd already gotten to know one another really well, really fast—a level of knowing that can come only from dissecting a human cadaver together, as we all did throughout our first year.

"What specialty are you going into?" is also the medical school equivalent of asking a couple who has just started dating when they are going to get married, or if they've just married, when they plan to have a kid. In this case, it suggests there is always something coming up that we will need to compete for. In a room full of type A, achievement-oriented people (myself included), we knew that this well-worn icebreaker was not meant to stoke our enthusiasm for medicine or encourage us to bond. It was enticing us to one-up each other, a game we easily played because we had been doing it most of our lives.

Someone started off, inevitably, by announcing that they were going to go into dermatology, followed by a chorus of people pinning their hopes on a future in anesthesia or ophthalmology, everyone naming the specialties that are hardest to get into, the ones that require the highest test scores, and those that have the least number of spots available nationwide.

No one ever dares to say out loud that they want to be a pediatrician or an internal medicine doctor, even though most of our class will likely end up going into those fields. While they are critically important and meaningful professions, in the medical school classroom, composed of self-created winners and losers, these fields are not prestigious enough. But if this game failed to "break the ice," the intensity of the competition in the room would do the trick.

As everyone gave their answers, I listened intently, growing more and more uncomfortable. Then again, in medical school I was uncomfortable most of the time. A large part of me felt I would always lag behind my classmates because, instead of majoring in biology or chemistry, I entered medical school as an undergrad anthropology major.

Then, the person to the left of me spoke up. "I'm Andrew, and I've always wanted to be a neurosurgeon."

Of course he does, and of course I have to go after him.

I took a deep breath and exhaled as I somehow blurted out exactly what I was thinking: "My name is Jessi Gold, and I'm not even sure I want to be a doctor."

The room was silent, except for a few awkward laughs that were attempts to pass off my comment as a joke. There was a tangible sense of fear that my doubt was contagious.

While it was the first time I had said it out loud, it certainly wasn't the last.

Ask any of my loved ones, and you'll hear that long before I decided to become a psychiatrist, I was the empathetic-listener type. I was always the friend people called for a willing ear and, sometimes, brutal honesty. You could say that I'm the consummate empath, and as such, it wasn't a stretch for me to answer the implicit essay question on every med school application: Why do you want to go into medicine? Like everyone else, I answered: To help people. It's the obvious answer, isn't it? Selflessness makes applicants appear genuine and caring—attributes most of us would want in a doctor. Plus, for many would-be doctors, including me, it's a genuine motivation.

Truthfully, though, I've always been a sucker for positive reinforcement, and not just the kind that comes with being a good person. As much as I or any prospective doctor might want to help others, it's tough to ignore the achievement and prestige perks that come with being an MD. Both motivations exist, even if we don't write "For the prestige" on our applications.

I wasn't necessarily born an overachieving, highly competitive science nerd, but I started young and took to the challenge enthusiastically. I trace my achievement-oriented roots all the way back to my parents' decision to have me start school a year earlier than I was supposed to. They like to joke that it was because I was reading at age four and really needed to "get out of the house already." But in all honesty, back then, I just loved learning. I liked memorizing a poem every week and practicing it in my head. I liked completing summer reading challenges, devouring as many books as I possibly could so that I could win first prize and go with the school librarian to Pizza Hut for a free lunch. I even liked taking tests, mostly because I was good at taking them.

Each semester, I'd write down my academic goals, and later, when I joined the swim team, I'd add my swimming goals, too: Get all A's, Make Junior Olympic times in my best events. I then taped the list of goals to our family's fridge. My two older brothers and my older sister did, too. I'm not sure how or when the tradition started, but I'm sure having similarly high-achieving parents didn't hurt—an international expert psychiatrist for a father and a mother with a master's in public health from Yale.

And the list worked. If I met my goals, in addition to praise I'd get some kind of reward—a toy, or even on one occasion a pet bird. I quickly learned that getting an A meant receiving praise from my parents, which was sometimes tough to do, as the youngest of four. Meeting my goals also made me feel good about myself—proud and self-confident, as if all my energy, drive, and efforts had been validated. I wanted to keep it up.

Soon, success in school became enmeshed in my identity. *Smart kids do well in school*, I thought. *You're a smart kid, so you do, too.* My dad used to joke that our best sport, as the designated "nerds" of the family, was test taking, and we competed with a number 2 pencil. I agreed, and I really, *really* liked winning.

I should point out here that my definitions of *winning* and of *doing well* were—well, *are*—warped. What I wanted to be was perfect.

No one told me I needed to get all A's all the time. They didn't have to. Achievement was the oxygen my family breathed, and I absorbed it by watching everyone else, but mainly my siblings. That's also how I learned what would get me in trouble with my parents (lying); what the coolest TV shows were (*Friends* and *Sex and the City*); how hard it was to get into a good college; and what precisely a *good college* meant.

By the time I was in middle school, two of my siblings were already at Ivy League universities and were members of their respective swim teams (one became captain). I'm aware that substantial privilege comes with being able to say that, but in my world it also created an extremely high standard to live up to.

It's perhaps not shocking, then, that my goals at the time (according to a page of the autobiography I wrote for a class assignment in fifth grade) included swimming in the Olympics and getting into an

Ivy League school because, to quote the great Elle Woods in *Legally Blonde*, "What, like it's hard?"

As I progressed through the years, though, getting a good grade no longer felt fun or exciting. It felt like an expectation, a foregone conclusion. As the tests got harder, I got harder on myself. If there was even a chance I might get a B, I freaked out and asked for help from a friend, a teacher, and sometimes a hired tutor. One time, I even stayed an hour later in a school entrance exam because I thought I would miss one math question. Yes, I was *that* girl.

By the sixth grade, I got kicked out of the classroom and into the hall more times than I can count for maybe a bit too enthusiastically waving my hand in the air as the teacher asked, looking straight at me, "Does anyone *else* know the answer?" Sometimes, instead of calling on me, the teacher would tell the class the answer, and I'd get so mad I would say something obnoxious (hence, the kicking out). Put simply, I was a know-it-all. But more specifically, I learned how big emotions got me into big trouble, and to be successful, I needed them to stop.

My childhood New Year's resolutions written in a diary from even before that time—"Don't cry," "Don't make faces," and, my personal favorite, "Don't talk about nothing for no reason"—make it clear that, early on, I was on a mission to not feel things so deeply, or at least not show that I did. It was my attempt not to be, as my family had dubbed me, the *emotional one*. I didn't want to stick out, even in my family, for that trait. Instead, I wanted grades and achievements to draw the attention to me.

I later learned to limit my emotions for a bigger purpose—becoming a doctor.

2

IN MARCH 2020, I woke up to an email that changed everything. Subject: Alternative Operations. It sounded almost military in nature, and that alone increased my anxiety.

If truth be told, I'd been glued to my inbox for the last few weeks, ever since the "novel coronavirus" appeared in the United States. Now, with every ding of my email, there was another pronouncement, another restriction, first to the states we were allowed to travel to (Subject: COVID-19 Travel Policy), then new rules for our own quarantine (Subject: Important: New Policies in Response to COVID-19). I locked on to the tiniest amount of guidance to somehow gain control of the endless stream of previously unimaginable information coming at me at full speed.

This particular message, addressed to all employees in the university and hospital system, started by emphasizing these "unprecedented" times, then laid out a plan to reduce disease spread by limiting who should go to work in person. Since, thanks to video software and telephones, my work as an outpatient psychiatrist, specializing in treating college students and healthcare workers, doesn't require I physically be in my clinic, I qualified to stay home. It didn't matter that I'd never before used video software to see patients, or that I tend to struggle to keep my focus when talking to patients on the telephone for anything beyond a quick question. According to this email, by definition, I was apparently "nonessential."

Now, even saying that word *nonessential* still makes me uncomfortable. As a medical student, I got used to trudging through blizzards to get to a shift, sometimes through snow so deep some of my classmates literally skied to the hospital. I learned that because hospitals are always open, physicians should work according to the Postal Service's creed: "Neither snow nor rain nor heat nor gloom of night . . ." would keep us from seeing to our duties, or in our case, our patients.

That work ethic—showing up, always—is even more crucial in an emergency. Doctors work through hurricanes, run toward the hospital after mass shootings or terrorism events, and wait to help, even if patients don't come (as I remember happened with me and many of my fellow medical trainees during the Sandy Hook shooting).

On an airplane, including traveling to or from vacation, those in the medical profession never totally let down their guard, knowing that if a flight attendant announces, "Is there a doctor on board?" then we must spring into action and help. True, a psychiatrist might not be anyone's first choice (or tenth) in these situations, but if there are no better qualified healthcare workers available, I help—and have helped multiple times. We can't even turn off at home around our family and friends. Beyond being the people who are constantly asked for medical advice or possible recommendations for care, medical professionals have told me about performing CPR on a parent or the Heimlich maneuver on a friend. Suffice it to say, I have always felt essential.

Not this time, though. Now, I was supposed to stay on the sidelines, setting up shop in my home office, protected by my computer. My medical residency—the four years of psychiatry-specific training I did after my four years of medical school—didn't prepare me for this. I don't know that anything could have.

My schedule for today is packed, as it has always been, with eight patients in less than five hours. Patient number four is currently between me and my lunch (and bathroom) break and is a new one, who, according to his chart, is thirty-six years old, self-identifies as Latinx, and prefers to be called Luke. I double-click Start Video Visit and see a shoulder-length, curly-haired medical resident (a.k.a. doctor in training) wearing a white coat, with his name embroidered on it just above the large colorful logo representing another hospital in the area. Underneath, he is wearing a collared shirt and a bow tie—basically what stock photos of doctors show them wearing. Well, that is, except for the tattoo I can barely make out, which is just under his right coat sleeve. I'm intrigued and will definitely plan to ask him about it, because encouraging tattoo stories are some of the best ways to get to know a patient (I mean, the tattoo is permanently on their body for a reason!).

But not just yet. First, I need to introduce myself, as I do in all my new visits. "Hi, I'm . . . ," but he puts up his finger and stops me in my tracks. I'm instantly taken aback and feel a bit confused, even nervous. Still, I stop talking as he looks behind him, then back at me, then behind him again. His finger is still up, and I wonder who he's looking for and, most important, if he's in a private place to talk.

It hasn't been that long—only three weeks—but I'm learning that there's something less controlled and more chaotic about telehealth visits than there is in office visits. A virtual appointment can take place in a car (moving or stationary), a bathroom, or a bedroom; patients have seen me while they smoke in a park, eat in a cafeteria, or play with their infant. I'm no longer surprised by what pops up on my screen at the start of a new visit; the surprise is even part of the charm. The problem is that psychiatry visits are supposed to be controlled. There's safety in control. That's why many of us share a collective image of a therapist's office: plain white walls, a piece of framed peaceful art, and a couch. The trust comes in the monotony. The room is always there waiting, protected, for patients to disclose their feelings.

With remote visits, though, the person a patient wants to talk about is often in that same room, or at least in the same building. At this point, I've already had patients use the Chat function to type in things about their husband or child they want me to know but they can't say out loud; "I don't even love him anymore" or "We've been fighting nonstop." I've been trying to adjust to this new situation, but privacy and safety are core to what I do, and my telehealth skill set feels a bit wobbly.

Luke finally puts his hand down, and I think we're ready to start. I almost start talking again, but he begins fidgeting with his head-phones, taking them off and putting them back in. One earbud falls out, he grabs it, and he puts it back in his ear. It falls out again, and he scrambles yet again to put it back in. Luke seems frazzled. I feel like I'm watching a scene not meant for my eyes.

I mouth, "It's okay if you can't use them," and he nods but goes right back to trying to get the headphones to work. I wait.

Without his uttering a word, I've learned a lot about him already. As a psychiatrist, I'm trained to observe a patient's appearance, walk, mannerisms, and degree of eye contact. I also notice details like whether they're tired or have otherwise been taking care of them-selves, or if they're so depressed that, from the looks of it, they've likely just rolled out of bed.

These observations create something called the *mental status exam*, which is similar to a physical exam but instead of listening to someone's heart and lungs, or looking in their ears, the psychiatrist is observing the whole of the patient. We then use it to help come up with a diagnosis. In fact, sometimes acquaintances worry that I also do this in social situations. Once people learn I'm a psychiatrist, some immediately say, "Are you judging me?" and laugh. It makes me feel defensive and uncomfortable, but I usually employ humor by saying, "Do you want me to?"

Observing Luke for the past five minutes or so, I can tell he's nervous—at least about being here with me. It's clear he seems fear-ful of someone's noticing or hearing our visit, and perhaps of dis-covering he's seeing a psychiatrist. It makes me wonder what "being here" means to him and what he thinks it would mean to other people. I make a mental note to listen for the answer, and when I get to know him better, I will try to ask these questions directly; doing so right now might seem invasive.

Truthfully, I admire Luke for coming to see me at all. Research shows that perceptions about mental health in medicine start early—even if a medical student doesn't think getting help for their mental health is a weakness, they worry that other people will view it that way. They fear being judged by everyone: supervisors, peers, people evaluating their residency applications, and even their patients.[1] Of course, their own cultural and family beliefs about mental health—and for Luke, mental health in men—come into play here as well, compounding the effects of medical culture. As a result, they often don't get help at all, with medical students more hesitant to seek help than others their age in the general population.[2] And if they do finally get help, as Luke is doing now, they try to hide it.

Being in medicine and taking their cues from others around them teaches students and trainees to feel shame about their own mental health. There's an unspoken rule that if doctors are having emotional struggles, they should keep it to themselves. This is just one part of what is known as the "hidden curriculum," a term coined in 1994 by researchers F. W. Hafferty and R. Franks,[3] which refers to the implicit teachings of medicine—the things doctors learn outside the classroom. How a doctor should feel or not feel and what to say about it (or not) are absolutely embedded in that curriculum.

However, ignoring mental health problems does not make them go away. Just look at the statistics. Long before COVID, multiple studies across physicians and physicians-in-training showed the prevalence of burnout to be as high as 50 percent at any one point in time.[4] And 28 percent of residents experienced depression, a number significantly higher than the general public.[5] We also knew that this can, and does, have devastating consequences, including high rates of suicide in physicians and nurses.[6] In fact, in a large national study of more than

4,800 physicians,[7] nearly 1 in 15 had thoughts of taking their own life in the last year, which exceeds the number among workers in other fields. Mental health outcomes are an occupational hazard in healthcare.

Still, doctors and doctors-in-training don't often talk about these things. Our emotional suffering is medicine's dirty little secret, and it's perpetuated, in many cases, by fear. Residents tell medical students about the person who got help for a mental health crisis and lost their license, or who took time away from their residency program and wasn't allowed to return, or who received fewer opportunities or lower grades as a result. People who ask for help are the subject of gossip and are judged. While thankfully many training programs now offer well-being lectures to normalize the conversation, and access to affordable, confidential mental health treatment (like me!) as part of accreditation requirements,[8] these services unfortunately go underutilized. In one study, despite access to mental health care, only 24 percent of residents who felt they needed help actually got it.[9] Of course, time and money are enormous barriers to seeking care as well, but improving access can do only so much when the culture itself prevents physicians from asking for help in the first place. The issues are systemic.

In a sea of white coats, no one wants to stand out because of their mental health. We prefer to be noticed because of our test scores or surgical skills. We want to appear perfect. It's no wonder Luke is so nervous about someone's catching on to what he is doing, talking to me.

And Luke is, finally, talking, earbuds in place. "Hi, sorry. Can you hear me?" he asks nervously. I nod. "I think everything is working now. I just wanted to make sure no one could hear us."

"It's okay. I want to check before we start; even if no one can hear us, are you in a place where you feel you can talk freely?"

"Yes, I think so." His body language suggests otherwise. With arms crossed, he hasn't yet met my eyes through the screen. His concern is also contagious; I begin to worry that someone will barge in on his session. But I move forward and ask, as I always do in my first visits, "I can tell very little from your chart, so it would be better to hear it from you. What brings you to see me today?"

Luke takes another look behind him. When he is sure the coast is clear, he starts talking. "Well, ever since COVID started, I can't stop thinking about how I'm going to get infected or that I'm already infected." I nod, again hoping he will keep talking without prompting. "I know a lot of people worry about that, especially people who work in medicine, and it's a real possibility that I could get COVID working with patients, or even from the social worker on our team who just went out for quarantine because she tested positive. But the actual risks aside, my thoughts about getting the virus have just become so extreme."

"What do you mean . . . *extreme*?" I echo, using a technique in question asking that I like, which is asking for clarification by using a patient's own words.

"I mean I'm at the point where I don't want to go into a patient's room because *I might get COVID and die*. That's what I keep thinking to myself, over and over. If I have a new patient, I will sit in the work room and basically hit Refresh on my computer, over and over and over, to see if their COVID test results are back. I can't make myself stop refreshing. Then, before I go into their room, I'm so afraid of getting sick that it takes me three times as long as anyone else to put on my PPE [personal protective equipment]. I've watched all the videos about how to put it on and have taken notes. I understand how to do it, but I feel the need to double-check, then triple-check . . . that there is no way COVID can get through what I am wearing. After all that, and doing everything I can to protect myself, when I leave the patient's room, I'm still convinced I've somehow gotten infected . . . and I can't seem to shake that fear."

I'm not shocked by any of this. The fear Luke is embodying is in line with what a lot of my healthcare-worker patients are experiencing. Before COVID, most healthcare workers went into work without thinking about the risks to themselves, as those risks were minimal. There might have been a few jokes about getting some stomach bug on a pediatrics rotation (I'm guilty of the jokes and karma of getting the bug!), and everyone gets flu shots every winter (it's mandatory, for one thing). But it was never common to worry about dying or infecting our families. Now, some healthcare workers aren't sleeping at home so as to keep their families safe, while others have died in the very hospitals in which they worked. In that sense, Luke's fears are very much justified. Yet his concerns go beyond "typical worries." For one thing, they're nonstop, and they seem to be substantially affecting his day-to-day life. As a psychiatrist, that's where I become concerned.

I try to be validating, but I struggle to find the right words: "That seems like it would make your workday really . . . challenging." I try not to assume how people feel about something by using stronger words, like *hard*.

"Absolutely. Everything takes me longer and causes more stress. Even washing my hands. I've started to wash them more often, for more than the length of 'Happy Birthday' [the song we learn counts as a good handwashing technique in med school]. It's like I have to sing 'Happy Birthday' three times to even walk away from the sink. I'm incredibly sick of that song now."

"What would happen if you didn't wash your hands, or at least didn't wash them three times?"

"Well, I'd get COVID and die. I know that sounds irrational, but I just can't stop thinking about it." He's speaking rather quickly, which might be an indication of his anxiety, or maybe it's just a desire to get this session over with. Or maybe it's both.

"Honestly, at this point, I'm really worried that I will not be able to do my job."

There it is—the answer I've been trying to get to. This is why Luke is here today and why he is here *now*. It's something I try to discover with all my first-visit patients: Why now? A person can have an extensive mental health history, or multiple recent triggers, but I need to know why they came today and not three months ago. I now know Luke is truly worried that his symptoms will impact his ability to practice medicine. Even for someone so clearly uncomfortable about getting help, the prospect of not getting help finally became worse.

Luke is far from my only healthcare patient who hesitated to get care until they couldn't wait a minute longer. In a sense, it's remarkable that Luke came in at all. According to a Kaiser Family Foundation survey, 17 percent of healthcare workers reported that the reason they thought they needed help, but didn't get it, was that they were afraid or embarrassed to seek care.[10] And in a study of first-year residents, 57 percent were so concerned about confidentiality that they opted to not seek help at all.[11]

Clearly, Luke is a product of a medical culture with a long history of being like this. As he talks, I think of all the people who never come see me, no matter how much they are suffering. People who have emailed me for referrals off the record, or who have direct-messaged me on X (Twitter) but have never set up an appointment during which I might take notes. I've had patients who wanted to pay in cash for visits or medications so there would be no evidence of our meeting.

Similarly, I have psychiatrist friends who've been asked to prescribe medications for alternative uses, like Wellbutrin (bupropion) for "smoking cessation" (it does work for that), when the real problem was depression. And when filling out short-term disability paperwork for healthcare-worker patients, I've been asked to put down items like "hip injury" or "fibromyalgia pain," as opposed to depression. I obviously can't do that, but their concerns are real: What if people knew?

Given the patient population I treat, I even have colleagues who've come to see me for mental health concerns who later ignore me when we pass in the halls or attend department meetings, as if they couldn't have met me any other way but as their doctor. These same people have no problem going to an OB-GYN or a urologist at their hospital and talking to that person the next day at work. But mental health visits cross the line. They are *too* private.

I'm glad that Luke, despite all this, is taking the first step and is here with me, asking for help. I really hope I don't scare him away as I gently ask him to share more of his concerns about missing work, though I have a good idea of what's coming.

"Yeah, I mean, I'm a resident, so my schedule changes all the time. One month, I'm working in the ICU or on cardiology; the next, I'm on general medicine. Any of these patients can be a COVID patient, so it's not like I can say I won't see anyone with COVID for whatever month. That's not a thing anymore. I also don't have that kind of power or flexibility."

He's right, I think. There is so little control in residency—something I remember vividly from my own residency. I know it also from having been chief resident, which meant in my fourth year of psychiatry training I was one of the people responsible for organizing the resident schedules, teaching, and often providing emotional support. I regularly think about what it was like when a resident was out sick or had to take time off for an emergency, and I had to find someone else to cover their shift. We had residents prepared to come in during these situations, but they never *wanted* to be called. I had to be the bearer of bad news, yet hearing their reactions (often anger) made me feel even more hesitant to ever call in sick myself.

As I look at Luke, I want to go off on a tirade about residency, but I stop myself, knowing that could make our visit about me. Instead, I ask, "Is this—the fear of infection—something you've experienced before or has it only been since COVID?"

In a first visit with a patient, I want to understand how that person got to where "here" actually is. To do that, I ask a laundry list of questions to be sure I don't miss anything. I always want to know about someone's past psychiatric history, as well as their current symptoms (which could include everything from hallucinations, to suicidality, to substance use). I then go on to ask about family history, medical history (including current medications and allergies), and social history (the person's support system, education, and employment). To patients, this process can easily feel like an information-gathering overload, but it's the best way for me to figure out how I can help, so I try to be as thorough as I can.

Luke pauses to think and replies, "I mean, *maybe* little fears here or there bothered me, but nothing like this. Nothing my mom or teachers mentioned, outside of me being 'very organized.' I guess in medical school, sometimes I'd read about a disease, then briefly worry about getting it, but doesn't everyone? It would be really short-lived though, and this keeps going on and on."

He's right about a lot of medical students thinking they have whatever diseases they're studying at the moment, a phenomenon that even has its own name: medical student syndrome. Somehow I avoided ever having it myself, but for Luke, those experiences are by no means diagnostic.

I know I need a better measure for how his symptoms are different now, so I ask for more information on how they are impacting his life. This is one of the best ways to measure symptom severity for all mental disorders, and it helps me understand if someone is just "a little anxious," for example, or if their anxiety is so intense they can't go to work or function. Mental health runs across a spectrum, and these kinds of details help me better clarify where someone sits on it. So, I ask, "How much time in your day do you think these thoughts or actions, like washing your hands or checking your protective gear, take up?"

"Too much. Like, hours?"

"If you had to be specific?" I gently prod him, since an objective measurement can really help me characterize him now and also enables seeing progress in the future.

"Oof. I don't know, maybe ten hours or something?"

"That's a lot of time and energy you could be using for . . . I don't know . . . sleeping?" I say, trying to lighten the mood. He cracks a small smile.

"This may be somewhat surprising, but what you're describing sounds a lot like obsessive compulsive disorder (OCD) to me. I'm sure you remember it from medical school, but here's a quick refresh, since I think we don't do a great job of teaching mental health in general. To be diagnosed with OCD, you need to have obsessions, which are recurring and persistent thoughts or urges that are intrusive and cause distress—like your concern about getting COVID and dying—and/or compulsions, which are repetitive behaviors or mental acts that someone feels they need to perform in response to their obsession.[12] To me, your handwashing sounds like a compulsion you're doing to try to minimize your distress over getting infected, or maybe even to prevent it from happening at all. It also sounds like you're doing things in a patterned way, singing 'Happy Birthday' and checking three times everything from the chart to your PPE. This is usually because if you checked it fewer than three times, the thing you were concerned about happening—in your case, getting COVID—could still happen. The third time is basically the 'charm' to soothe your obsessive thought."

Luke looks both confused and shocked at the same time. "Oh, wow, I'd never thought about that. I mean, my boyfriend and family have said I'm *obsessive*, but OCD? Really?"

"There are so many different symptoms and presentations of OCD. That makes it hard to get a full picture, especially because we tend to use the acronym colloquially—'Oh, I'm so OCD'—when people just mean they clean a lot or are particular or organized; it's like they told you when you were little, which probably felt like a compliment. It's honestly hard to see yourself as having something if your image of it is nothing like your experience."

"What you're saying makes sense. But what can I even do about it? It's not like I can just stop everything and . . . unless you're saying . . . wait, do you think I can work like this?"

My insides start to rumble with anxiety when he asks this question. I don't like telling people they might have to interrupt their careers, even for a little bit. Especially when that career cost a lot of time and energy. (Luke is approaching his last year of three years of medical residency and plans to apply for a fellowship, or for additional subspecialty training, likely in hematology-oncology, for another three years soon.) It's a sacrifice to establish that career and it has become an integral part of his identity. That's something I totally relate to.

"I think that's a long conversation, and honestly, the answer depends on how safe you feel doing your job. Obviously, if you feel that what you're experiencing is affecting your patient care right now, absolutely you need time off." I pause and note that he looks concerned. Gently, I say, "It sounds like time off to get treatment—start therapy and a medication—could be helpful. At a bare minimum, it would allow you to remove yourself from potential high exposure to COVID, so you can start to heal."

I notice Luke's facial expression hasn't changed, so I stop my argument and instead try to validate what I think he's thinking, "But I also know taking time off in residency isn't easy."

"Yeah . . . I'm sorry," he says, a bit irritated. "I just can't imagine taking time off right now. Everyone would have to cover for me, and they'd all think something was horribly wrong with me and I don't even want to tell them what's wrong, because they'd judge me for it, and I don't know how I could make up the time . . . and . . . I'm the first person in my family to go to college, let alone med school, and I'd let everyone down. . . ." He is speaking so fast he can't even finish his sentence, and I have trouble completely following his thinking. I can see just from looking that his thoughts are spinning. They make mine spin, too.

Well, at least until they land on one overarching word: *burden.* That's because every schedule change, every need, every human experience affects everyone around you in healthcare, particularly as a resident. No one likes to be a burden. Keeping quiet and keeping on feel like the better options. *Been there, done that.*

Luke takes a deep breath and continues. "I just worry about burdening my residency friends, who honestly have enough to deal with right now. So, since I'm not a risk to patients, and I have insight into my thoughts being abnormal, which I remember is good and could help me know if they get worse, if I don't stop working right this minute, what would your plan be for me going forward?"

"I think ideally you would go to therapy and start a medicine. Then we'd monitor your symptoms at work and see if you do need to take time off in the future. The therapy I think you should do is called exposure and response prevention (ERP). It's an evidence-based treatment that has been shown to reduce obsessive, compulsive, anxiety, and depressive symptoms." [13]

Luke stays quiet, so I continue. "It's actually a pretty cool therapy. Basically, you gradually expose yourself to your fears—for you, germs—until you get more comfortable with them. It's the opposite of that old show *Fear Factor*, where they dumped people with a fear of snakes into a giant tank of snakes. Instead, you might first imagine a snake, then maybe you'd be around a toy snake, then maybe you'd go in the same room as a snake, and so on and so on until eventually, the feared object becomes boring instead of anxiety provoking or scary. It's based on habituation, which is a natural process whereby we stop responding or paying attention to a trigger after repeated exposure."[14]

I pause my mini lecture to make sure he's still following. He nods and politely says, "Oh, I remember learning something about that."

"I realize that it sounds kind of terrifying, too, so just know that feeling is normal."

"Thanks for saying that." He smiles. "I'll look into starting that for now, and will call some people." I offer to give him a list of names of therapists who specialize in ERP and OCD, which he happily accepts, but I feel guilty that I don't have a way to get him seen faster.

He then pauses and looks at me as if he is worried about my re-action to what might come next. "Also, you can save your taking-medication spiel for now. I'm not ready for pills. That feels like too much."

I don't react. I come from a place where I assume people are skeptical and hesitant about medication, especially psychiatric meds, and it's their right to be as patients. I respond, "I *completely* understand. I've seen medications really help a lot of people, but I also understand hearing all of this information is a lot. . . . So, I'm not pushing you *at all*. If you want, and absolutely no pressure, I can just write down the names of the medications I would recommend, for you to think or read about."

Giving people time to read and think is something I believe in doing in my practice. It helps patients know what they are getting into and it allows them to figure out their questions before they talk to me again. People with medical backgrounds who experience anxiety are especially likely to want to do research, and then they'll come back with specific questions. That's totally okay with me. I believe if they then do eventually choose to go on medication, they'll feel more in-volved in the decision. That matters.

Luke doesn't protest, so I take my cue to add, "Something to keep in mind about medicine is that sometimes people with OCD need a higher dose to really target the symptoms—sometimes more than the maximum daily dose. And, a word of warning I wish I didn't have to give, but just know that there are a lot of antipsychiatry websites out there, and they *really* do not like medication. Take what you read on-line with a grain of salt, and try to stick to expert sites where you can. Or, bring back things that you read and I can help talk you through them before you take them as facts."

He reassures me he'll use UpToDate (the most common peer-reviewed quick reference site for doctors) or look things up in a med-ical textbook, rather than just reading whatever Google shows, adding, "Having those medication names could really help."

I immediately start typing the names of two different types of antidepressants into our chat. I give him the option of sertraline (Zoloft), a selective serotonin reuptake inhibitor (SSRI), and clomipramine (Anafranil), a tricyclic antidepressant often used in OCD.[15] As I type their names, I add, "Those aren't the only options, but those are two popular ones and a good starting place."

We say goodbye, and I know that even though I didn't prescribe a medication, I helped Luke today. He stayed the whole visit and told me what was going on with him. It might have been the first time he ever told anyone how he was feeling. He was by no means comfortable, but still, he talked.

This is progress. We all need to start somewhere.

3

I ENTERED MEDICAL school absolutely certain of one thing: I didn't want to be a psychiatrist, like my father.

I'm sure someone like Freud could come up with a deep therapeutic reason for why I didn't want to follow in my father's footsteps. Or, maybe I could ask the surgeon who belittled me as a medical student and asked, "Are you going to go into the same field as your daddy?" as he looked down at me awkwardly holding a retractor during an operation. But all I can come up with is that my dad's shoes are big, and I was afraid to try to fill them. It felt like a goal I couldn't achieve or a competition I simply wouldn't win. And I don't like losing.

Don't get me wrong, though, I respect my father immensely. He is an expert in his field of addiction and is a researcher with hundreds of publications to his name. A lot of people at my medical school knew him personally because he had trained there. One time, I went to an addiction psychiatry meeting, and someone saw my last name on a name tag and asked me if we were related. I tried to say no rather vigorously, but apparently in protesting, my mannerisms, humor, and sarcasm made it even more obvious that I was my father's daughter.

Avoidance, to me, felt like the safest tactic. Since I was fascinated by the brain, I tried my hardest to veer toward neurology instead. In medical school, I joined the neurology interest group, sought out neurology mentors, and even did neurology research. But I kept find-

ing myself feeling happiest when I could talk with patients and hear
their stories. Even when I was supposed to focus on a procedure or
make a tricky diagnosis, I just wanted to pull up a chair and talk to
the patients about their lives.

I remember, during my internal medicine rotation in my third
year of medical school, I was taking care of a patient named Rosa, a
seventy-five-year-old woman with worsening chronic obstructive
pulmonary disease (COPD), a progressive lung disease. Every morning at 6 a.m., I went into her room and asked, "How are you doing
this morning?" She would smile, seemingly not minding that I'd
woken her (unlike the patient who taped a note to the hospital door
that read, "Do not bother patient until 6 a.m., especially med students"). Without skipping a beat, she always said, "Good morning,
Cookie."

I found her greeting endearing; it made me think of my grandmother, who like Rosa also loved red lipstick and talking about her
grandchildren.

One morning, my medical team got a page: "East Pavilion 5-512.
New onset chest pain. Please come evaluate."

"That's Rosa's room," I said out loud to no one, as the team had
already picked up their pace to climb the stairs to see her. As we ap-
proached, I heard the sound of her screams—feeble but urgent.

Once in her room, I locked eyes with Rosa, who looked nothing
like she had a few hours earlier, when we had joked with each other.
Now she was crying and sweating, almost childlike in her discomfort,
begging for someone to listen to her. In fact, she was screaming for
someone to listen.

The residents scrambled to complete the typical diagnostic steps
for chest pain, pulling down the top of her gown and adhering the
EKG machine's electrodes to her sunken chest to ascertain her heart
rhythm. Someone came to draw blood so as to see if she had elevated
troponin, a protein that spikes when the heart muscle has been dam-
aged. Someone else ordered an X-ray of her chest. No one noticed

that Rosa was upset that her chest was exposed. No one made any effort to cover her up.

I was in the corner of the room, out of everyone's way, watching the scene unfold like following a checklist of "what to do for chest pain." At each step, the residents told me—I was the only medical student in the room—what they were doing. They wanted to teach me something, even in the controlled chaos of the emergency, and I wanted to absorb it all. But I couldn't stop looking at Rosa's face.

Suddenly she coughed, which provoked an ear-piercing "*Ay, dios mio*," as she looked at the ceiling, presumably praying to God. She spoke English fluently, but now the only words that came out through her pain were in Spanish. Sometimes there's safety and comfort in a person's native language.

I felt a pit in my stomach, and I took it as a sign to do something. Ignoring the unspoken rules of medical professionalism, I ran to Rosa's side, making sure not to get in the way of the *real* doctors. Then I asked her permission to hold her hand, and she nodded okay. I also re-arranged her robe so that her chest was not so exposed, again being careful not to interfere with the team's maneuvers. After that, I squatted down to her so we were at eye level, and I said in a quiet whisper, "It's going to be okay."

Rosa replied, "Thank you, Cookie, for caring about me."

I instantly felt defensive of the team, knowing that they cared, too, but as I looked around the room, I realized Rosa's point. It wasn't as if there was something wrong with these doctors, or this well-regarded teaching hospital, or that anyone was doing the wrong thing. They were all trying to save her life. But in the chaos of the beeping monitors and the diagnostic steps, they forgot that it was a human being whom they were saving.

I couldn't stop seeing the person, in this case Rosa. I wondered if, in the future, I would be able to distance myself as my colleagues seemed able to do. And at the same time, I wasn't sure I wanted to do that.

Maybe that's what drew me to psychiatry. Not only is it a field in which patients feel seen, but within it I felt seen, too.

I remember on the first day of my psychiatry rotation I walked into the offices of the Veterans Affairs hospital to find my name listed on the door; even better, I had my very own desk.

This may seem trivial, but as a medical student I often had to fight to be able to use the one available computer or had to alternate with nurses at the nursing station. Not having a space of my own made me feel like an afterthought—or even a burden. Being referred to as "the med student" didn't help. But in psychiatry, as soon as I saw my name on the door along with the "real" doctors, I felt like a person again. For the first time in a few years, I could see myself being happy in medicine.

And even though I'm happy, I know I don't necessarily fit the image most people have of a psychiatrist—something I'm always conscious of, whether I'm with my patients, meeting new friends, or on a dating app. Many people assume psychiatrists are old white men in sweaters, who see patients for a single visit, ask no questions about their life, and just give out medication. Basically, that they are glorified prescription-drug dealers. But for me, that couldn't be further from the truth. Yes, I do primarily see people for medication management, despite having trained in therapy, as all psychiatrists do. But that is about where the similarities end between what and how I practice and those popular notions of psychiatry.

For one thing, I'm a millennial, though I look even younger than my age. I was carded on an airplane while sitting in an emergency exit row when I was twenty—the minimum age requirement is fifteen years old—and I still sometimes get asked for my ID when I order a drink at a bar. I'm also a female with long curly hair, and I tend to talk to my patients exactly how I talk to my friends—that is, informally and in real time. The only exception is my sailor's mouth in conversations with my friends. I rarely curse in my appointments, unless I am echoing a patient's use of a word. For example, a patient might say, "Today really fucking sucks." And I might reply, "Tell me more about why it fucking sucks."

My tone of voice is the same one I use in normal conversation. I don't have a "therapy voice"—that calm, sort of lowered radio-show tone that many of my peers seem to adopt. And this voice tone was a purposeful decision on my part. I've always found it hard to be anything other than who I am. I also find that my patients tend to relax and feel more comfortable with me when I seem real to them—like someone who could be a friend.

It's not that I don't choose my words with care, but even when I'm explaining medications to patients I tend toward informality, talking about side effects in understandable ways and staying away from medical jargon, if I can help it. For instance, to explain the most common antidepressants—selective serotonin reuptake inhibitors (SSRIs)—I might stick with something along the lines of "the drugs make more of one of the chemicals in your brain that make you happy" rather than "there is a mood-related neurotransmitter in the brain called serotonin, and the drugs are thought to work by blocking the reabsorption of it into the neurons." Or, instead of my listing all the side effects and the percentage likelihood of experiencing each, I'll say something like, "Some people say SSRIs make them gain weight, and that could be because when someone is sad and anxious, they tend to eat a lot, or it could be an actual metabolism change." I want to make sure people understand what they can expect from medications and that they feel comfortable asking me anything about them. Though there is not a lot of evidence on this, there have been several studies suggesting that physicians who have a warm, friendly, reassuring manner are more effective than those who are formal and don't offer reassurance.[1]

Perhaps somewhat obviously, I might not use this same tactic with a patient who is a healthcare worker, as the person might feel as if I am talking down to them by not using the jargon. Instead, I typically ask if they even need an explanation or remember and know it themselves, giving them space to admit that they, like me for some (okay, most) other medical fields, do not remember the details and need a reminder. I also have a touch of impostor syndrome when seeing my peers as patients, and I don't want them to mistake my being informal with being unqualified.

Still, I've been known to joke around or make a pop-culture reference or two during a session. One time, a patient was talking about a breakup and said, "We are never getting back together"; I absolutely could not stop myself from referencing Taylor Swift's hit song, replying, "Like ever." She laughed, but also made fun of me. She said, "Did you *really* just quote Taylor Swift? . . . Seriously, who are you?" I didn't mind her comeback because it not only lowered her stress level but also strengthened our relationship—as studies on the use of humor in therapy have shown.[2]

Of course, not every patient will like or respond to humor, and it shouldn't be used in every situation. I'm mindful of that. In certain instances, a patient might interpret humor as trivializing or minimizing their problems.[3] That's unhelpful, since recognizing a patient's problems as valid is often key to effective therapy. This is likely why, when my own therapist asks me how I feel about an incident in my life or at work, and I sarcastically respond, "It was SO fun," she is driven to remind me that sarcasm isn't a feeling. "Tell me how you *really* feel," she'll urge.

I struggle to turn off the humor completely, however, and suspect that's one reason I feel drawn to certain patient populations, like college students. I also think it's one big reason why they're drawn to me. They are often a little goofy, a lot of the time.

With humor or not, for an empath like me, practicing psychiatry can also take an emotional toll. Though the actual hours in the field are "normal" compared to the twelve-hour medical shifts in other departments and the overnight and weekend calls, the lesser hours don't quantify the weight of the conversations that take place in session. As psychiatrists, we are often the first people our patients tell their stories to, and we hear about some of the darkest aspects of life, including trauma, abuse, loss, or grave illness. Sometimes our patients even end their lives, with approximately half of all psychiatrists experiencing the suicide loss of at least one patient.[4] Many trainees who are drawn to psychiatry because of the better work-life balance it offers don't often consider this emotional toll. It doesn't mean psychiatrists don't enjoy what we do, but the impact of that toll is significant and can't be ignored.

The fact that so many psychiatrists choose the field because of their own mental health struggles, or because of struggles in their own families, only compounds the weight of other people's pain. Sometimes, the heaviest emotional burden is to bear witness or to hold space for someone else's story. To do my job well and be someone whom people can trust, I need to care. I need to be truly empathetic. I need to be raw and available. But being empathetic in a world with so much pain and so much hate sometimes feels unbearable—as if I'm being eaten alive. There's no clocking out.

I think often of a quote by poet and author David Jones: "It is both a blessing and a curse to feel everything so very deeply."[5]

4

I SOMETIMES STILL get anxious before seeing a new patient. I think it's the not knowing what lies ahead that gets to me. I've learned to try to calm myself by obtaining more information, but sadly this can happen only on the rare occasion when I have time to prepare for a visit—like today.

In these few extra moments, I quickly review someone's chart, paying particular attention to whether they have seen a psychiatrist before or if their primary-care doctor referred them because of a particular reason ("anxiety" or "trouble concentrating" come to mind). I also glance at their medication list and play a game of *spot the psychiatric medications*, past and present. Seeing multiple types of antidepressants, for instance, might mean the doctor before me kept trying new medications, or even adding them, when an old one wasn't working. Once I had a patient on five different drugs that started with the letter *L* (Lamictal, Lexapro, Lorazepam . . . you get the picture). Jokingly, I asked him if his psychiatrist was practicing *Sesame Street* medicine and today was "brought to him by the letter L." He laughed, but really it wasn't funny because it meant I had to figure out which of his medications to keep and which to take away or change. Not knowing which meds in the mix are working is probably one of the harder tasks in my job.

Sometimes, though, the person has never been seen at our academic institution, in any department, and there are no notes, no medications—nothing to go on; when that happens, I'm flying blind. Other times, the background I have makes me worry even more. Like, if they've tried ten or eleven medications earlier and nothing has worked; then I start to think I won't be able to help either. It's hard in those instances to feel confident I can find the one remaining medication that might miraculously work. If I'm honest with myself, in cases like these I worry that I won't be good enough, that someone's problem will be outside my knowledge base, and that maybe I'll fail—which doesn't feel like an option when failing can worsen someone's mental health.

Ultimately, I push all those feelings away and see the next new patient anyway. Like so many of my doctor patients, I'm good at compartmentalizing.

This time, the new face on my screen is an anxious-looking twenty-year-old woman named Naya. She's wearing a purple sweatshirt emblazoned with the name of her college, which she isn't currently at because of COVID. Like so many students around the country, she went home for what she thought was going to be a week of spring break but she couldn't go back. I guess I kind of did that, too.

Unlike Luke, Naya didn't fill out the self-identifying demographic information on the chart, so I start by asking her how she identifies. People often get race wrong by just assuming, and it is important to clarify and ask, especially in psychiatry when identity can be so essential to presentation. She tells me, "Black."

Medicine used to place race at the beginning of all our clinical presentations and notes ("This is a 70 y/o Chinese woman who presents with trouble breathing"), and in psychiatry it often was mentioned in the appearance section of the mental status exam. But I've since had mentors explain how this tradition is biasing and the literature agrees.[1] I've slowly unlearned this older approach, but I mention Naya's race here because she did.

"Oh, wow, I don't even know where to start," she says, sounding somewhat overwhelmed at my "What brings you to see me?" question. "Do you want to know *everything*?"

"Most things," I respond with a smile. "Try telling me what you want me to know, and then I'll ask you specific questions if I need to know more. Don't worry, I'm good at filling in the gaps."

"Okay." Naya looks away nervously and starts to fidget with her dangly earrings, which are just barely noticeable behind her intricately braided hair. I nod, encouraging her to talk. I try not to make it obvious that I notice her fidgeting, but there aren't many other places for me to look other than at her face on the screen. I make an effort to focus my attention to the area behind her, where on the wall I can see pictures of what I assume are her friends and posters of her favorite movies. One advantage of telehealth is that I can learn other details about a person because I often see them in their own home; it gives me a small window onto their life.

The viewing is not mutual, though, because hospital management has advised us not to let patients see our homes on the screen. All that's visible to Naya is a gray background with my hospital's name in the corner. Still, it's possible she might know more about me than I let on in this initial session, simply by doing what many of my patients do before their first visit and looking me up online. She might have seen my Instagram or X feed, or read something I wrote about mental health that appeared in the popular press. Even though I love doing public advocacy, I worry that a patient might develop unrealistic hopes for an appointment with "the psychiatrist they saw on TV." My office wall with its fancy degrees from various Ivy League schools only compounds those beliefs—or biases. I'm genuinely afraid I won't live up to their expectations, or perhaps most significantly, my own expectations.

If Naya could see the walls behind me, she'd glimpse the covers of Broadway playbills, from *Hamilton* to *Cat on a Hot Tin Roof*. These are mementos I've collected from shows stretching back to childhood. I wonder if they would make her like me more, humanize me a little bit, but this visit isn't about her knowing me.

Naya continues, "So, last week, I was supposed to take my MCAT and instead I ended up in the ER. That sounds dramatic, but it *was* dramatic." Her speech is picking up speed.

"I was late to the exam," she continues, "and I honestly have no idea how that happened because I planned it all out days before. I looked up the route, and even drove to the testing center at the same time as my test would be the week before, so I'd know how long it would take to get there with traffic. On the day of, I set five alarms, like 6:00, 6:05, 6:10 . . . you get it."

More than you know, I am thinking, as I recall the two alarms I set just to make sure I woke up for work this morning.

"And I was on time . . . until I wasn't. There was an accident on the highway, and I was late. It was out of my hands, I guess, but all I could hear in my head as I ran into the testing center was 'You will never be a doctor now.'"

I shift my body to show I'm listening (not so easy to convey on a computer screen) and notice I'm getting anxious for her. I start thinking about my own experience taking the MCAT, or any other standardized test, and I feel nauseated. Just like I did right before I threw up during the ACT exam in high school (don't worry, I made it to the bathroom).

My anxious reaction with Naya is a textbook example of *counter-transference*, a fancy term for a psychotherapist's internal and external reactions to a patient. Typically, these reactions are influenced by the therapist's own history, conflicts, and vulnerabilities.[2] The reactions aren't harmless, though, and can negatively affect therapy and whether it works.[3] As a result, we learn to manage these issues by being constantly aware of our own reactions to patients and our feelings about them. We are also taught to use this information—our own reactions—to deepen our knowledge of a patient and help us guide their treatment.

Psychiatry was the only specialty in medical school in which attending doctors (those who have finished training and are practicing medicine) regularly asked me, "How does that patient make *you* feel?"

Answering that question can be uncomfortable. It means breaking down the barriers between our work selves and our other selves, and between doctor and patient. It means acknowledging the fact that not only are we human but we also are humans with issues of our own that can crop up while we work. It likewise means we can be affected by our patients, sometimes in intense ways.

For example, in training, I noticed I would become annoyed, or even angry, when seeing a particular type of patient. These were the ones who most pushed my buttons. I realized over time they were patients who expected me to fix everything for them, as if I had a magic wand, instead of acknowledging that medication has limits or that they might need also to see a therapist and delve deeper into some of their stressors. It took me a while to realize that when a patient feels helpless and expects me to "fix" them, that helplessness gets transferred to me—and I don't like feeling helpless. At the same time, I know I can't fix everything, which makes me feel imperfect, even ineffective. And that triggers my own self-worth issues. Understanding all this about myself, I now know that if I'm angry or annoyed with a patient, I can let that feeling inform—and not interfere with—my care of them.

Of course, awareness is just the first step of many, which is why it's good for people in mental health fields to be in therapy themselves. This is so much so that most psychiatry and therapy training programs encourage it, and some even give credit for it. As Carl Jung, the famous Swiss psychiatrist and early pioneer of psychoanalysis, once said, "Knowing your own darkness is the best method for dealing with the darknesses of other people."[4]

Naya finally stops talking to take a big breath, as I check the time on my computer screen to see if I need to begin interrupting her so as to get some specific, targeted questions answered. Managing the time during a visit is always a bit challenging, but is even more so when patients have a lot of emotional content to get out. Graceful navigation means giving them space to talk, then getting all the data needed—it is often an art, especially when I'm also trying to gain their trust.

It's only been about ten minutes. *We're okay,* I think to myself, which is good, as Naya jumps right back into speed-talking and telling her story. "When I got to the door of the test room, I started to bang on it. This woman came out and first told me to be quiet, because testing was in progress, which really pissed me off, and then, once I told her why I was there, she said I couldn't take the test because I was too late." She takes another deep breath.

"I couldn't even get out the words to explain that I had been held up because of an accident, but I don't know that she would have cared. I got so emotional that I really started to have trouble breathing, and then my hands were tingling and my chest hurt, and I started sweating. I've never freaked out like that in front of anyone before. And I was super-embarrassed, too. I needed to sit down because it felt like I was going to die. I've read that women experience heart attacks differently, so I wondered, *Could I have a heart attack about the MCAT at age twenty?*"

"That must've been really scary," I reply, noticing that as she relayed the events, except for the fast speech, she had little emotional reaction and was mostly making sure to get out all the facts. It was almost as if she had completely disconnected from her feelings about it all, which, judging from her story, were obviously strong. *It's a form of unconscious protection against something traumatic and painful,* I think to myself. *I have to be careful not to make it worse.*

She shifts in her seat, back and forth, fiddling again with her earrings. Each time she moves, I find myself wanting to move, too. That restless contagion is usually a sign of just how bad someone's anxiety is—and Naya's is palpable.

"Those sensations didn't stop, even after, like, fifteen minutes," she continues. "So, I called my mom who works at the university to come pick me up. She could barely understand me, through the hyperventilation and sobbing, but luckily, she knew where I was because we'd talked about it for months. But when she got there, I still couldn't really calm down. I tried to walk a bit with her outside, but it didn't help. I really thought I was having a heart attack, so we decided to go to the ER."

"I can totally understand how you got to that decision. What did they do or say there?" I ask, knowing the answer from so many other patients' experiences, but wanting to hear her tell it so as to better understand how it all affected her.

"The doctor there did a bunch of tests to make sure my heart was fine, but only after we asked multiple times. Initially, he said, 'I bet you're having a panic attack.' I was really annoyed by that assumption. It felt like he was saying, 'It's all in your head.' My mom agreed, so we pushed him to do all the tests anyway."

This happens way too often. When patients and their families try to advocate for themselves the way Naya and her mother did, they are often ignored—or worse, they are labeled as difficult, or made to feel as if they are. This all also happens much more frequently with Black patients. In one study, Black patients had 2.54 times the odds of having one or more negative descriptors (like "agitated" or "refused") in their electronic health records, as compared to white patients.[5]

Naya's story also brings to mind the many patients who show up in my office angry about being told their problems are psychological. And honestly, sometimes the way they've been treated by the medical system has actually *caused* their psychiatric symptoms. Existing biases about a person's gender and race are also a part of it, compounding the stressors or negative treatment. For example, Black patients are more often given lower triage scores (indicating urgency) in an emergency room,[6] and are less likely to be referred to diagnostic testing and major therapeutic procedures, even after adjusting for insurance status and disease severity.[7] I can imagine some of this had occurred to Naya and her mother in the ER, and simultaneously it likely triggered other experiences they've had with healthcare in their past.

Of course, the ability to make quick judgments is often necessary when a doctor is figuring out the steps to take to save a life. But, as helpful as that skill is in an emergency, it can lead to mistakes. A common mistake is believing someone's symptoms are due to the most obvious answer (a.k.a., a horse), instead of something more rare or outside the box (a.k.a., a zebra). An assumed diagnosis can then prevent a doctor from even considering alternatives or running needed diagnostic tests, a concept called *representativeness error*.[8] This, too, is worsened by implicit and explicit biases about race or gender.

In Naya's case, however, all her heart tests were fine. "The doctor came back to say his hypothesis was right . . . that what I was experiencing was definitely panic," she tells me. "That only made me hate him more and really not even want to listen to what he had to say. But then they gave me an IV with meds in it to calm me down, and it helped, so I tried not to let my feelings take over. They also gave me a handout about panic attacks, and I have read a lot more about them since. I wish I didn't agree with him, but . . ."

The perception of her doctor's arrogance and potential biases aside, Naya's description of what happened to her is about as classic as it gets for a panic attack, nearly straight out of the *Diagnostic and Statistical Manual of Mental Disorders* (*DSM*, for short). The *DSM* is a handbook created by the American Psychiatric Association in 1952. It contains descriptions, symptoms, and other criteria to help diagnose mental health disorders. The manual is revised regularly, with input from hundreds of clinicians (the latest version, *DSM-5-TR*, came out in March 2022). Periodically, new diagnoses are added, or the criteria for a disorder are changed, or a diagnosis no longer considered a mental disorder is removed, as homosexuality was in 1974. While I don't see the *DSM* as a bible of psychiatry, as it's so often described, nevertheless it does provide a framework for questions and diagnostic understanding, even if there's a lot of overlap between diagnoses. Real life is seldom that clear-cut.

According to the *DSM*, to be considered as having had a panic attack, a patient needs to show four or more symptoms from a list of thirteen. Naya had six symptoms: palpitations, tingling arms, sweating, shortness of breath, chest pain, and fear of dying. Plus, like so many of my patients with panic attacks, she ended up in the ER. In fact, 18 to 25 percent of all patients who present to the ER with chest pain are actually experiencing panic and not a heart attack.[9] Still, when a new, scary symptom comes on, it's hard to fathom it could be caused by your brain. And when an ER doctor diagnoses those symptoms as panic so quickly and so definitively, especially before ruling out other medical conditions—something the *DSM* says has to happen—patients can feel defensive and dismissed. I'm just happy Naya kept an open mind, read the pamphlet she was given, and even did her own research. I'm also happy she's here.

I tell her that I agree with the panic diagnosis, adding a long-winded explanation of the brain and body connection in an attempt to validate her symptoms. There's a right way to tell people their physical symptoms are being produced by psychiatric causes, without negating their experience. Empathy helps.

I think about the time back in high school, when I had to get out of the pool during a big swim meet where I was doing the 200-yard butterfly, because I was having a horrible asthma attack. For many meets after that, anytime I was doing that event, if I got winded—likely because I was swimming as fast as I possibly could—I freaked out that I couldn't breathe, which made everything worse. I was convinced it was asthma every time, and I got out of the pool a few more times mid-race. But, really, it was a vicious cycle that my brain had created. I told myself to *stop being crazy and overreacting.* That had been my family's advice. "You're putting too much pressure on yourself," they'd say. I had a chance to help Naya in a different, more effective way, I hoped.

"Did those symptoms happen just that one time?" I ask, knowing that it's unlikely an experience like hers will be a one-and-done.

"After the shock wore off, I thought I'd be better . . . but I've still been really on edge, constantly worried, and I have had one of these episodes every day since. None has been as big as the first one, but they just keep happening, and they're exhausting. I can't think about anything else when they are happening, or for hours after. And I certainly can't get anything done, like studying."

"Do you notice any triggers, like events or conversations?"

"Well, at first, they seemed totally random," she says slowly. "It was as if I had no control over anything. Then I noticed the panic was happening whenever someone talked to me about the test, or my next steps, or I tried to study for a science class, or even think about studying for the MCAT again. I mean, I still have to take the test at some point. I just don't know how I can possibly do everything I need to do right now, because literally my whole life is a trigger. But I can't afford to miss class or to not study, or not take the test. I just need to take it and score highly so I can get into a good medical school."

I allow myself a friendly little laugh. "Is that all?"

She smiles and laughs, her deep brown eyes actually looking into mine for the first time.

———

I know first-hand how many mental health stressors prospective medical students experience when trying to become a doctor. First, there are the undergraduate course requirements: a year each of biology, chemistry, organic chemistry, and physics, all with labs, plus a year of math. Some schools have additional requirements, like English/writing and biochemistry.

Most of these courses feel disconnected from clinical medicine, which might be because the curriculum was defined in 1905 by the Council on Medical Education of the American Medical Association; unbelievably, little about it has changed since then.[10] Plus, none of these required classes are easy, and each is more competitive than the last. Given that the average GPA of matriculating medical students is 3.74,[11] the pressure is off the charts to do well in challenging classes where everyone is competing on a curve for an A. In one 2001 survey, 68 percent of former premed students pointed to their low grades as a major reason for dropping out—with 78 percent mentioning organic chemistry as the single course that most affected their plans. Women and underrepresented minorities (URM) were especially likely to mention this reason.[12]

And getting good enough grades is just the first hurdle. Medical school applicants are expected to complete relevant extracurriculars, such as shadowing physicians and conducting research, not to mention taking that pesky MCAT. The highest possible MCAT score is a 528, with a 132 on each of the four sections.[13] For those accepted to medical school, the average MCAT is as high as 511.9, so it's no surprise that Naya believes she needs to do exceptionally well to become a doctor. The kicker is that, study after study has shown that grades and MCAT scores have no bearing on a doctor's clinical performance or patient satisfaction with their care.[14]

Some students describe the whole getting-into-medical-school process as a series of steps or hurdles; others call it a culling or weeding out. Part of that view is based on just how competitive the field is to begin with and the mentality it creates owing to such a limited number of available spots. According to the American Association for Medical Colleges (AAMC), in 2021, 62,443 people applied to medical school but only 23,711 were accepted,[15] or about 38 percent. Naya's anxiety about the MCAT was indeed directly linked to her future. Just like mine had been.

I don't tell Naya about my own experiences as a premed, though. Psychiatrists are supposed to be blank slates, not people with their own experiences (or social media profiles, for that matter). As such, I have become adept at slipping some of my stories or coping skills into my visits by saying "I have a patient who," when I'm actually talking about myself. However, a study of therapists at a university counseling center[16] found that clients who were treated by therapists with more self-disclosure (meaning the therapists talked about themselves more) had lower levels of distress from their mental health symptoms, and reported liking their therapists more. Perhaps, like many ideas that started with Freud and then were perpetuated by others, we should take the blank slate concept with a grain of salt.

"It's all a lot to deal with," I tell Naya, wanting to say more, but worried that we don't have enough time remaining in the visit. I then change course, using a conversational tactic I've learned can steer patients away from even the most emotional topics. "Not meaning to cut off the conversation, which is super-important, but I want to make sure we talk about treatment. Did the ER physician talk to you about how we treat panic?"

"He said to make an appointment to talk to you."

I smile. "Well, that's a good start. I obviously prescribe medication, but not everyone needs medication for panic. A lot of people benefit from trying to understand their triggers in therapy and learning to use coping skills when they start to notice an attack coming."

"Yeah, I think I would consider that, and I would appreciate some names. But I'm a bit more nervous about medications, not because I don't think they can help, but because I don't know that I can handle anything new in my body right now."

I nod, understanding her concerns and wondering how much more detail she can absorb today. "I totally get not wanting a new medication, especially right before your test. I'm just trying to help you have this panic interfere less in your life, especially since you are having attacks every day and are having difficulty functioning. So, let me just ask you this: Do you think it could help, for now, to at least have something to take as needed, in the moment you're having an attack?"

"Hm. It might. Even to just know it's there."

"Kind of like a security blanket?

"Yes! Exactly!" She looks at me a bit skeptically, "What medication do you mean, though?"

I reply, "I'm not thinking of giving you the same medication they gave you in the ER, if that's what you are wondering. I honestly think you would be so mad at me if you took something that made you tired and interfered with your ability to study. What I'm thinking about is a medication called propranolol, which is a beta blocker used to target the body's fight-or-flight response to stress in the moment. In higher doses, it's used to treat high blood pressure or a fast heartbeat, but someone figured out it had a pretty good effect at calming people's nerves if taken in a lower dose, such as before giving a speech, taking a test, or doing anything stressful. Sometimes celebrities on the red carpet will say something like 'I took my beta blocker' and that is what they mean."

"Oh yeah, yeah, I've heard of that."

While she mulls it over, I think about how, after I struggled with test-taking anxiety during the first of my three-step board exams for medical licensure, my medical school dean said, "You should've just taken a beta blocker." I didn't even know that was a thing then. I hoped to catch Naya earlier than my experience.

"I think I'm willing to try that," she tells me. "I kind of hope I never have to use it, but I'm willing to have you prescribe it."

"Honestly, I also hope you don't have to use it," I reply with a smile.

Then we both wave awkward goodbyes to each other from screen to screen, and I kind of feel as if I've been looking into a mirror, talking to my younger self.

I hoped to help her the way I wish I'd been helped.

I'VE BEEN PRACTICING telehealth for over a month now, and as much as I miss being in the room with people, I am getting used to it. I have a set routine whereby, with no commute, I can wake up a bit later and still have time to shower and get ready, even if "ready" means dressing in comfy pants and my Ugg slippers, with a Zoom-appropriate shirt. As someone who used to immediately change into sweats after work, I like this new definition of office attire. After I shower, I walk my dog, an eight-pound Maltipoo named Winnie (like Winnie the Maltipoo), around the neighborhood, a quiet suburb. Too quiet. I live in the kind of neighborhood where most people know each other by sight and say hi. But the pandemic has changed the community. Fewer people are out running or even walking their dogs, and when they are, they keep their distance.

After a quick breakfast, I settle down at my desk for a long day of patients. Winnie settles in, too, sitting behind me on a lounge chair that she thinks was put there expressly for her because of its proximity to the floor. Her constant company makes me feel less alone.

My first visit of the day begins at 8 a.m. On this particular day, there is a fifty-three-year-old self-identifying white woman sitting across from me, via the computer screen, who is named Megan. I am seeing her for the first time, and I can't help but notice how piercing her green-eyed gaze is—almost like a glare. I don't know what's behind the stare, but something about it feels both judgmental and inquisitive at the same time. I find myself hoping that she gives me the benefit of the doubt—maybe it will help that a friend of hers recommended me, and even emailed me to be sure I could fit her in.

Beyond the stare, I notice that her screen is a bit shaky, like she is having trouble getting what seems to be her phone (instead of a computer) to stay still while she talks to me. Being able to log in to a remote visit from a phone is nice, and accessible, especially for people with no time as is, but the computer app is a bit more functional to say the least. In between the roller-coaster visuals, I see a seatbelt and the back seat of a car. I'm pretty sure that means Megan is sitting in her car, though I hope she is not driving. She is also still in her scrub top, and I put it together that she must be in her hospital's garage, having just finished her night shift. Looking at her tired-appearing face, I can't help but think of my own night shifts, and how even with blackout curtains and an occasional Benadryl, I could never catch up on sleep during the day, eventually snapping at people and crying more easily as the weeks went on. I didn't envy her, and I knew what additional mental health stressors, and effects on her alertness and performance,[1] simply working the night shift can cause.

Megan drops her gaze, then pushes back her headband on her gray hair, which is in a messy ponytail. She has that cool color of gray—more silver—that every woman hopes their hair will turn so they don't have to dye it. In the dim light of the garage, the shadows beneath her green eyes are somehow amplified. When I look closely, I can see the indentations from her N-95 mask, which she has likely been wearing for twelve solid hours, a visible symbol of the added strain of the pandemic.

We banter back and forth a bit about the weather, and she responds to my getting-to-know-you questions with short, direct answers, like the efficient ER physician she is. She reminds me a lot of my mentors in the confidence she exudes, and also her unflinching seriousness. She wants to get to the point, and quickly. No dillydallying here. I simply want her to like me. I always feel that way about my patients, but there's something about Megan that's bringing it out even more. Maybe it's the fact that she's more senior, and thus triggering all my reactions to hierarchy, good and bad.

"So, how are you feeling today?" I try, and she replies with a terse "I'm okay." I don't know her well enough yet to tell her that *okay* isn't a feeling. For that matter, neither is *fine,* or *alright.* Besides, I know she isn't okay. For one thing, she came to see me.

"Tell me why you are here today." I try switching to facts, instead of feelings. Facts may be more in her comfort zone.

She takes a deep breath as if to answer, but before she can, she starts to cry. I'm surprised, but not shocked.

"I'm so sorry. I don't know what's wrong with me. I never cry," she says, between shallow breaths and slow-falling tears. "Seriously, I am so, so sorry. . . ."

She keeps trying to regain her composure, and every time a tear falls, she apologizes. Most of my patients do this when they cry, especially the women. It's as if crying is something they should feel ashamed of because it indicates they are feeling too much. I do it, too.

"I promise that crying is not a problem or something to apologize for," I say, trying to comfort her and normalize her experience. "In my office, crying is like *hello* or a handshake. If you can't cry here . . ."

She smiles a little bit.

I do, too.

Maybe that stupid joke worked, I think to myself, hoping she will now feel more comfortable in this virtual room with me. It's not like I can shift my body language (pointing my legs toward her or leaning closer) to better show I care. I also can't just hand her a tissue through the computer screen. Psychiatrists have few actual physical tools (my stethoscope sits on my shelf in case of emergencies), but tissues are absolutely one of them.

I think about the time in medical school when I became aware of their true value. I was on an internal-medicine rotation at a community hospital with a resident who was an empathetic teacher. My patient, June, an unmarried woman in her early seventies, had cancer, a diagnosis we had just learned from her scan. I had never seen someone get bad news before and I sure wasn't ready to deliver it myself. I was glad that my resident understood that and would be the one telling June as I watched and learned.

As my resident started to speak, it was as if June already knew what he was going to say, because she immediately started to cry. He paused, looked for the tissue box in the room, and brought it to her bed. He took one tissue out of the box and handed it to her, then put the box close, within her reach. He didn't keep talking; instead, he simply let her cry, being present with her while she did. The tissue was better than any pat statement I could have come up with. It didn't take a lot of time to grab the box, and it didn't divert the discussion, but it was a way of telling her that he was there. That her feelings were welcome.

Before that encounter, I had never considered how doing something so simple could mean so much to a patient. But studies have shown that small acts do matter. For example, compared with doctors who remain standing, patients whose physicians sit down in the exam room rate their doctors higher on measures of listening carefully and explaining things clearly.[2]

With the tissue offer, my resident showed me how to simply acknowledge someone's humanity. I wondered how I could replicate that through a screen, for Megan. I wanted to say, "If I was in the room with you, I'd hand you a tissue," but that sounded odd, so I just kept silent.

Megan sighed and continued. "Well, that started differently than I thought it would. I'm just so surprised by my crying. I mean, I came to see you today *because* I've been feeling so off and flat, even outside of work. I actually really don't cry. At least, I haven't in a long time. I remember a time when I did, but I don't anymore. It has been years, or even decades. Ha! That dates me a little."

"You haven't cried in decades?" I say, emphasizing her statement in part to make sure I heard her correctly, and also because I'm amazed by the number. "Can you tell me more about that?"

"Sure, yeah, I mean, the last time I remember really crying, I was in med school, in a room with this patient who was coding. I think it was the first time I'd ever seen a code," Megan continues. "I wasn't allowed to help because I was a student, but I could watch, which was maybe worse. The patient was a young woman in her thirties. She'd been in a car accident, and she died right in front of me. Someone said, Time of death, 21:30, and I heard the beeps of the machines stop and I looked around the room. No one said anything. There were literally no words, no change in facial expressions—nothing. I started to get that feeling that happens just before tears come, and I just ran out. Like, *ran* as fast as I could, out of the room and into the bathroom. I didn't want the rest of the team to see me cry, but a few of the attendings saw me running. They just looked at me and didn't say a word. They didn't have to. I got the message."

"And . . . what was that?" I asked.

"There's no crying in medicine," she almost whispers.

"Did someone actually say that to you?" I wonder out loud.

"Well, not necessarily that wording specifically, but not one of them talked about the death or the code. They just went on to the next patient, or worse, to lunch."

I don't say this to Megan, but I honestly wish people would just at least acknowledge our jobs are weird, and that what we see, like codes and death, isn't normal; it can be traumatic.

She continues, "There was also this one time in residency when my program director called me in for a feedback session after I'd been struggling with a hard few weeks of really sick patients. I wasn't crying or anything, I was just . . . off. And, she said to me, verbatim: 'I don't care what you have to do. Go home and yell at your family, kick your dog, or drink yourself to sleep, but you come back to work in the morning and pretend like your feelings don't affect you.'"

Holy shit, I think to myself. *No wonder she's struggling with her feelings.*

Like Megan, many healthcare patients I see have told me that their first code ended up modeling how they should act during powerful emotional situations in medicine, like witnessing suffering and death. Usually, what they learn is to not react at all. Subjective evaluations and criticisms, like the words of her program director, just help to cement what counts as "acceptable" emotions in medicine. But I wanted Megan to know that she could have feelings, and that the feedback she received wasn't okay. I decided not to bother hiding my reaction to her story.

"Whoa, that was . . . *something* to say out loud," I respond. And it is the truth. I have heard a lot of bad things said to people in medicine, but this one truly shocked me.

Megan looks up, defeated. "Yeah, whenever I think about it, I still can't believe she actually said that. She meant it, too." For a moment, she looks uncomfortable. "But it's not like that was just said to me. I've heard other people get gossiped about for their feelings or called 'soft' or had their abilities questioned. So, I got the message loud and clear."

It's extremely common for those in the medical profession to regulate their emotions. One study[3] found that 43 percent of physicians tried to control their reactions to intense emotions, particularly so-called negative emotions like anger or sadness. And this tendency only becomes more rigid the longer doctors practice. Studies[4] suggest that empathy declines over the course of medical school, while cynicism increases. Relatedly, as physicians advance in their careers, they get better at hiding their feelings by suppressing them or distracting themselves.[5]

Medical students and residents are taught, explicitly and by example, that "good doctors" are stoic. As a resident, I once saw a medical student get in trouble for bringing a patient flowers, and a surgeon patient told me about a trainee being reprimanded for spending a few free moments reading *Green Eggs and Ham* to a terminally ill child. It was as if they were supposed to appear empathetic to a point, but if they cared too much, that was crossing a line, or bad doctoring. Such displays of empathy and emotion even affect trainees' grades, which rather obviously made an especially big impression on us achievement-oriented folks. Attendings are more likely to praise and promote behaviors people outside of medicine might deem callous, like not showing emotion when delivering bad news to a patient and not showing any excitement for the good times. Rather than improving a medical student's interpersonal skills, like empathy and communication (or "soft skills," as I've heard them negatively called), the focus is on teaching technical skills and expanding medical knowledge.

Some of this is grounded in good patient care, of course. An unemotional doctor can more easily remain composed in challenging situations and support patients through them.[6] Heightened emotions can increase the risk of errors,[7] and affect interactions with patients in a potentially detrimental way, especially if they are unrecognized. For example, healthcare workers in heightened emotional states might interrupt their patients or change the subject more, or even have their decision-making affected.[8] In other words, minimizing the impact of our stronger emotions, including those triggered by the patients themselves, might be beneficial to patient care. On the flip side, the short-term coping strategies many doctors turn to instead of expressing what they're feeling—like compartmentalizing or using substances at the end of the day to help relax—can have long-term consequences on their health. A doctor who compartmentalizes might also be seen as callous or uncaring, and patients might be less satisfied with their interactions as a result.[9]

Perhaps there is an in between—one where physicians can recognize their emotions and feel, but they can also move on and do their work, and go to the next patient unencumbered. Maybe there is a time and place for feelings. Even if we are told otherwise, it certainly can't be nowhere and never.

———

Megan goes on to tell me that after being reprimanded by her program director years ago, she stopped letting her emotions affect her. "I took it on as almost a challenge," she says. "Now, I'm so used to not expressing anything that I no longer put myself in the position of the patient. My job is to be the doctor and fix the patient. Feelings aren't part of it."

I take this all in and weigh my next words carefully, as I really don't want Megan to feel judged for how she is now or how she used to be.

Slowly, I say, "So . . . it seems like you stopped showing your feelings to survive, because you're a product of medicine. For better or worse. And since you're here, maybe it has finally caught up with you? Maybe you're even a little worried that it isn't 'normal.'"

I say this because her lack of noticeable emotion brought her to me in the first place, even though it has been her demeanor for years. Maybe she never connected it all before now—where it came from and how it's affecting her. But unexamined emotions can make physicians feel lonely or lose meaning in their jobs, and they can also create feelings of hopelessness and anger. This can result in depersonalization, which tangibly can look like lacking empathy for or having a negative attitude about patients, or seeing them more like tasks or to-dos, instead of humans. This attitude can spread to colleagues and the workplace, and often leads a person to feel cynical or numb. Depersonalization is a symptom of burnout, but it may be related to other mental health disorders like PTSD, substance use, and depression.

Though I'm not quite sure yet, I start to wonder if Megan might be burned out. Studies suggest that beginning with medical school, burnout is common; a third or more of all physicians experience at least one of the three components of burnout, defined by the World Health Organization as an occupational phenomenon in 2019. This includes emotional exhaustion and lack of feelings of personal accomplishment, in addition to depersonalization.[10] That's a consistently higher rate of burnout than in other professions, including law or academia, which require similarly lengthy schooling.[11] Another reason is that emotion regulation is directly correlated with burnout.[12]

While burnout itself is not depression, or even something found currently in the *DSM*, it is a steppingstone toward it, and even an independent risk factor for suicidal thoughts.[13] It can be thought of simply as the impact of a stressful workplace or the difference between what you think work will be (for healthcare workers, helping people and teaching) and what work actually is (paperwork). I think one of my patients said it best when he described his burnout this way: "I used to be able to go into work and see the roses through all of the thorns, but now I only see the thorns. Are there still any roses?" That is exactly how burnout feels.

Megan's emotional numbness and decrease in empathy could be considered depersonalization, and a lot of her comments directly relate to the culture of medicine and how it has impacted her. However, I'm not convinced burnout fully explains exactly what's going on with her now, and I plan to keep digging deeper during our visit.

I guess I'll start with more observation, as we find ourselves sitting in silence on opposite sides of the Zoom screen. I sense she is taking in what I've said and thinking about how it applies to her. I'm just trying to give her space to process in peace. And, I really mean *trying*, because I absolutely hate silence.

To patients, a period of silence may feel uncomfortable or just plain wrong, as if the therapist is disengaged or doesn't know what to say next. In actuality, it gives the therapist time to observe and think, and gives the patient space to make the unconscious conscious (as we mental health professionals love to say).[14] Beyond that utility, simply being able to sit in silence is often acknowledged as an important step toward improvement for the patient, demonstrating growth in interpersonal interactions.[15] Perhaps the same is true for providers.

In residency, my therapy supervisor would tell me to practice not responding, to sit in silence, even past the point of my discomfort with it. But I would always crack before the patients did and I would ask a follow-up question or laugh uncomfortably. I'm honestly not good at silence as the patient, either. I don't like sitting with too many thoughts in my head, whether I'm alone or with my therapist. Or even now, with Megan.

As hard as I try, I'm still the first to speak. I ask, "Has compartmentalizing ever been an issue for you, especially in places outside of work?"

"Not often. But, sometimes . . . like once at a family dinner when someone asked me about work, I told them about one shift where a bunch of members of one family had died in a car accident, a lot of them kids, and everyone looked so surprised. Some even teared up. And, then there's me just telling the story like I was ordering a cheeseburger. I didn't even stop eating dinner. At the time, seeing their reactions, it struck me that maybe something was off with me. I wondered, *Is it abnormal not to react to these situations?*"

I nod, encouraging her to go on, as I can tell there is more there.

"Then, the other evening, it kind of all came to a head. I was at a play with a friend who is a nurse. Anyway, right at intermission, we're sitting there and suddenly behind us there is all this commotion and a scream for help, and we notice that someone is down on the ground. We run back there to help, but the person, who was pretty old, had already died. After that, the two of us went back to our seats and waited for intermission to end, so we could watch the rest of the show. Some people walked out, and others tried to move their seats. We were the only people who didn't look stunned, and we were actually excited to watch the rest of the performance."

"That must have been somewhat surreal. What was it like for you? How did it make you feel?"

Megan looked me right in the eyes, laughed, and said, "Did you seriously just say that? I felt okay, Dr. Freud."

I laugh, a bit awkwardly. Truthfully, when I hear myself ask that "How do you feel?" question, I feel a little ridiculous myself.

The question, of course, is the most clichéd a psychiatrist can ask, yet it's critically important. It moves the conversation away from a simple narration of facts and pushes it into deeper territory, toward every psychiatrist's favorite topic: emotions. The only other time I've felt I was being "classically psychiatrist" was when I caught myself with my hand under my chin, looking like I was thinking deeply. I was really just holding my head up because it hurt from being tilted slightly for five hours. I wondered if maybe that's the real reason the pose came to be so famous.

Still, I can't help myself from being the psychiatrist I am, so I keep pressing Megan. "But . . . it doesn't sound okay. How did you *really* feel?"

"Like I didn't belong. Or, that I wasn't processing things like a human. I felt like everyone in that theater was staring at me, but instead of that dream where I'm in my underwear, it was because I didn't seem to care that someone had just died, like I was heartless or something. I'm worried this is just how I am now."

"Do you feel . . . not like a human?"

"Good question." She pauses and thinks in silence again. She is better at this silence thing than I am. I hold my breath and count, and hope she beats me to speaking this time. *One, two, three, four . . .*

"I just mean, most people would have feelings about what we see every day at the hospital. Especially when it happens *not* in the hospital. Not feeling anything is protective in the job, for sure, and I think it's good sometimes, but maybe it isn't good *all* the time."

"That seems to be a valid observation. I wonder, though—has something changed to bring you here now?"

"Well, I guess I've been reflecting a bit more lately, with COVID. The ERs are weird because we aren't seeing a lot of people who don't urgently need to be in the ER. You know, the people with an ache or pain, or the ones who really should go to their primary-care doctors, but go to the ER because they don't have anywhere else to go. They aren't coming in right now, because they don't want to catch COVID. Instead, the ER is full with a lot of people who urgently need me, and

I like that part. I feel really useful and honestly enjoy my job." As she says this, I start to think this can't be burnout, as meaning and purpose at work are protective against it and she seems to have both.

She continues, "But if I told an ordinary person what I saw every day, and there's way more interest in what work looks like for me now than ever before as no one else tangibly sees COVID's impact like we do, they'd be shocked or appalled. I made the mistake of doing that with my best friend, and he did something *much* worse—he called me a hero."

I already know, from what so many of my patients are telling me, that the word *hero* is just adding pressure to everything health-care workers are experiencing.[16] Heroes run toward an emergency, no questions asked, and absolutely don't have space to feel. There's no "Wonder Woman Goes to Therapy" episode, though maybe there should be.

"Do I dare ask you about your feelings on *that* word?"

She smiles. "It's just . . . No one acknowledges that any of us might have feelings about all of this. And being thought of as heroes makes us hide them even more, if that's even possible. I'm just trying to get by, and mostly put my head down and work. I just know there's more to me than this flat workaholic."

I think about the best way to help her work in the way she has become accustomed and at the same time find her feelings. I ask, "Do you have any ideas as to how to figure that out? How to find that part of you, again?"

"Well, I was hoping you did, preferably in the prescription variety."

I smile somewhat solemnly. "Will you hate me if I tell you that I don't think there's a pill that can fix your emotionlessness? That, at least right this minute, a pill isn't going to quickly make them reappear?"

As I say this, I think about how there are a few misconceptions about medications, but a common one I've seen among my physician-patients is that a prescription can fix symptoms that are bothering them, like sadness, or fatigue, or poor concentration, so they can get right back to work. Most of them actually want a medication more than they want to get to the root of the problem through talking (and more than other patients with fears of medication). They don't like talking about themselves. Yet as I often tell patients, "There's no pill that can 'Eternal Sunshine of the Spotless Mind' all your stressors away so you are just back to yourself."

Also, not everyone needs medication. Though some people believe a psychiatrist will hand out drugs whether a patient needs them or not, I believe there is a time and a place for medication, but there is also a time and a place to wait or talk with a therapist first. As is the case with Megan.

"But if medication isn't the answer, what does that mean for me?"

"I think you really need to keep getting to the root of your emotions in your life, and in work, through talk therapy." I see her visibly squirm on the screen in response to that plan. "And then come back to me if you don't think it's helping, or if you feel you're getting worse."

"Oh, man, I have to *talk* about it?"

"Yes. Is that uncomfortable?"

"Totally. I think today, with you, is the most I've talked about myself and my experiences in years."

"And how has it been?" I ask, hoping she'll say that she felt heard and safe, and not scared away from help seeking.

"Uncomfortable. Not because of you, but because no one really asks me about *my* feelings. And I certainly don't think about them myself."

As it turns out, as health professionals, being able to care for others does not mean we take time to care for ourselves or acknowledge our own emotions, especially during a crisis like the pandemic, when feelings are scary and big, and seem as if they could actually break us.

"I'm glad I asked, then, but I also hope I'm not the last."

6

___

I SUFFER FROM the same affliction as so many of my patients. I call it the "But I'm still doing well in school" mindset, comparing all the things in life that we're doing against academic or career achievements. No matter what else we're experiencing, or how bad we feel emotionally, if we are succeeding in work and school, we must be doing fine.

For my college students, this translates to waiting months, or even years, to see me because they are still getting good grades. It doesn't matter that they haven't left their rooms or seen their friends in weeks, or that their only nourishment is takeout foods. If their grades are good, they're good. The same goes for high achievers at work, except that presentations and performance reviews take the place of grades.

It's funny how, for so many, school and work can be the last things to suffer, even as they are suffering, going through the motions that enable them to "succeed." The thing is, that kind of success is an inaccurate benchmark of well-being. Yet, it's exactly why I delayed asking for help for the very first time in college. I simply didn't think I *needed* it.

My reluctance was compounded by the fact that no one else I knew was in therapy. Back then, in the early 2000s, therapy wasn't as talked about (or, dare I say, as trendy) as it is now. This was especially true in the highly competitive premed academic circles in which I traveled. The curves on the tests and the scarcity of spots in medical school tended to bring out the worst in people. To win the competition to be a doctor, I needed to have no weaknesses and needing help for my mental health would absolutely count as one.

But I couldn't deny that I was sleeping more, going to class in sweatpants every day, and getting angry at my friends over the smallest things. I also cried a lot more easily. These were signs of depression, but I didn't call them that. No one did.

I don't remember the exact tipping point, but like so many of my patients and friends, I got to a place where I had no choice but to take action. Maybe it's because I started to skip class, and that scared me—it might affect my grades. Whatever the reason, I finally made an appointment at the student health center to see a counselor. My expectations weren't high, but at least the help was free. It may sound unbelievable, but even with my dad being a psychiatrist, the decision to see someone felt huge. I believed in its effectiveness—just not for me. I had a habit, even then, of feeling that others deserved more nurturing and leeway than I did.

During my intake at the counseling center, the therapist asked me every question I ask now in my initial appointments with new patients. I didn't make it easy for her, though. I was guarded and protective, and I worried about what she might think of me. I wanted her to like me. I wanted her to say I was fine. So, without being conscious I was doing it, I minimized everything.

"What brings you in?"

"I don't know. I just feel . . . off."

"How so?"

"I guess I'm sleeping a lot more and a bit moody."

She didn't dig too deeply into that, but she kept running down a checklist: No, I'm not suicidal. No, I don't hear voices. No, I don't have a mental health history, and neither does anyone in my family. No, I've never taken medication before.

I didn't lie, but I never offered up more than she asked for. She was a stranger who didn't deserve to know things I hadn't yet admitted to myself. If she'd prodded a bit, I might have given more details, but she didn't.

As we neared the end of the fifty-minute visit, she paused and looked at me, and I waited for her to give me a diagnosis or tell me something she had noticed. Instead, she pursed her lips and said, "Thanks for coming in. Based on what you've told me, you don't qualify for on-campus treatment. Here is a list of therapists in the community."

I grabbed the list from her as I processed what she had said. I felt angry and confused, but also a bit excited. That's probably what happens when you know deep down there's something wrong with you, but you don't *want* something to be wrong with you. It's vindicating, but at the same time it doesn't feel good.

"What do you mean by that?" I asked.

"Well, you aren't sick *enough* to need to get treatment on campus."

Sick enough? I thought. *Who does she think she is, making a decision like that? Doesn't she know how hard it was for me to get myself here? This is why people don't ask for help.*

I wondered who actually was sick enough. *Did I need to be suicidal? Would I have made the cut, then?* I almost asked her those questions, with righteous indignation, but I was too ashamed. *There's no way I would tell her everything in a first visit,* I thought.

I wouldn't expect a patient of mine to tell me everything on a first visit, either, especially someone who had never seen a therapist before. She should have known I needed more encouragement, or at least another appointment. I deserved better.

"We have limited providers here, but if you want to talk to someone, you can connect with someone off campus." *Right, because I want to go through this whole thing again,* I thought to myself sarcastically. I knew the added barriers of needing to drive somewhere and to pay out of pocket were not going to make those next steps any easier. And what if the farther away, more expensive person also turned me away?

I left the office still feeling a bit stunned and not sure what to do next. Given that I hadn't wanted to go in the first place, I wondered if maybe I really *didn't* need help. Maybe she was giving me a stamp of approval to continue on exactly as I had been doing. *Your grades are fine. You are fine. You aren't that sick.*

Luckily, I didn't completely give up on therapy. I stuck with it, even though I made an appointment with an outside therapist who tried to blame my parents for everything that was wrong with me, like a shrink in a TV comedy, and I hated her. Somehow, I tried again and found someone I really liked—someone whom I saw for the rest of my college years and into medical school. I then found someone new again, in residency.

Since then, I've seen a therapist on pretty much an ongoing basis. But the one I have now, Dr. Miller, is different from the rest—special, even.

You would think that as a psychiatrist myself, I'd be able to come up with a good reason for why that is. But there are things about therapy that are ineffable—that are all about chemistry, things that go beyond words. I'd go so far as to say that finding a therapist is like dating (minus the romantic stuff), and when you truly click with a person, you just know. Dr. Miller *gets* me; she did from the very first sessions.

People always ask me how I find my therapists, as if I have some magical power or particular answer that might help them navigate the system. I wish I did, but the system is just as broken for the people working within it, meaning I find my therapists like most people do— through my insurance company or at the website psychologytoday .com. The latter is basically a large directory of therapists, complete with headshots and some basic details about insurance plans accepted and information about each person's way of practicing. I use it to weed out those who seem too different from me philosophically (too many mentions of feelings and crystals). I also use it to find someone who does the kind of therapy I'm interested in—psychodynamic therapy instead of cognitive behavioral therapy (CBT) or dialectical behavioral therapy (DBT), which involves more open-ended talking as opposed to learning specific coping skills or behaviors.

You might also think that because I'm a psychiatrist I can simply ask one of my colleagues for a recommendation, but even psychiatrists don't like to talk openly about their own mental health. Plus, when we do find someone we like, we're not inclined to share. No one wants to see the same therapist as their co-workers. I know from experience that this doesn't work out well.

This small world was particularly a problem during residency, since there were only a few therapists who took our insurance and didn't teach in the very same psychiatry department we were training in at in the medical school. As a result, a lot of the psychiatry residents ended up with the same therapists. One time, as I was going to an appointment, I saw, coming out of my therapist's office, a woman I'd clashed with at work. In my session, I brought it up. My therapist obviously couldn't confirm or deny this person was her client, but I still felt the need to ask. After that day, whenever I happened to mention the woman's name (which was often; she wasn't an easy colleague), I'd watch my therapist's face to see if she was taking sides. Even when her face stayed perfectly neutral, I'd judge her as not supporting me. It was a lose-lose situation, and mostly it prevented me from talking about this person at all. I honestly liked that therapist, but the situation made it impossible for me to be truly open with her. After a while, I dreaded going.

But as I said, I knew instantly that things would be different with my current therapist, Dr. Miller. I met her on January 30, 2020, a bit more than a month before the pandemic hit the United States. You might say the timing was fortuitous. Trust also doesn't come easily for me, but with Dr. Miller somehow I felt as if I could safely bare my soul from day one. I was especially proud that I didn't lie about a single thing. Yes, like most people, those of us trained in mental health sometimes lie to our therapists. And like most people, we don't like to admit that out loud. But even now, years after that first meeting with Dr. Miller, I haven't lied to her yet.

Though I refer to Dr. Miller as my "therapist" in conversations with friends and family, she is actually a PsyD, which stands for Doctor of Psychology. This means she has a doctorate, but instead of getting a PhD with more of a research focus, she chose to concentrate on clinical psychology for, on average, about six years. She also had to complete an internship, and by the end of that time, she and other PsyDs complete close to 5,000 hours of clinical work before seeing patients unsupervised. In other words, she has *a lot* of experience.

That's not always the case for people who call themselves therapists. Even as a mental health professional, I sometimes find confusing all the titles and types of practitioners. The truth is that many people can use the *therapist* title, including those with a PhD in psychology, a master's degree in counseling, a licensed professional counselor, a social worker, a marriage and family therapist, and a school counselor—though their years and types of training vary widely. Being able to afford, much less choose, a therapist is a privilege in the United States, not a given, but it's still important to do the research before picking what type of therapist to see. The more research you do, the greater the chance you'll find someone who matches your needs.

I wouldn't say I picked Dr. Miller simply because of her degree, but having that much training is certainly a plus in my eyes, especially owing to my own background. Psychiatrists are different from therapists in that we go to medical school; only instead of spending extra years training as a surgeon in the operating room, or as an OB-GYN delivering babies, for our residency we do an additional four years in different psychiatric settings. Because of this, we can (and do) pre-

scribe medications, though we still learn how to practice psychotherapy. Obviously, we spend less time studying and focusing on this
than does someone with Dr. Miller's experience, but we do see
therapy-specific patients during our training, including patients we
follow for the entire four years of our residency.

For each of those patients, we had supervision in groups with
other residents and individually with a therapist (not a psychiatrist!)
who went over our cases and discussed stuck points, as well as what
to do next. We also videotaped our sessions to get real-time feedback,
much like a football player reviewing films of their performance after
a game.

Because of my own training in therapy, though, I know that I can
be a bit annoying as a patient (or "client," as therapy patients are
often referred to today). There is a meta level to my therapy whereby
I can sometimes figure out what my therapist might be thinking
about me, why she chooses to say something, or what skill or technique she is using. I don't love that I can do this. I prefer when people surprise me—and more than once with Dr. Miller I have said,
"Oh, wow, I see what you did there." This makes me doubly appreciate her skill. Of course, she could have noted that I was a psychiatrist
on my intake form and turned me down as a patient. I'm lucky she
was up to the challenge of treating me.

I also tell people interested in my therapist-search process that
demographics mattered to me in my selection, as they do for a lot of
people. Some people might choose a therapist partly for their sexual
or gender identity or ethnicity (which is easier said than done). I se-
lected Dr. Miller for her gender identification (cis female) and age;
she is only a few years older than I am, which I prefer. I don't like feeling as if I'm being lectured to, or mothered, which has happened before. With Dr. Miller, our conversations feel more like two friends
talking, or at least, like a wise, slightly older sister talking to a younger
one. These are, of course, interactions I'm used to in my everyday life
(I have friends and a wise older sister!), but this relationship is differ-

ent. Mainly, it's one-sided by design, so when I talk about me, I feel less like a bad friend, or sister, or a burden. As a result, I'm more open to listening, learning, and sharing.

The immediate feeling of safety I experienced with Dr. Miller was surprising to me, and honestly has only grown over time. For therapy to work, meaning you make progress toward your goals and experience personal growth, the fit is everything. I talked about connection and chemistry earlier, but there is also a concept known as *therapeutic alliance*, which captures the collaborative relationship between therapist and patient, as well as their agreement on goals and their emotional bond. Study after study[1] has shown that there is a strong predictive relationship between therapeutic alliance and outcomes in individual therapy, and that it tends to remain consistent, no matter the treatment approach. The stronger the alliance, the more successful the therapy, period.

Liking Dr. Miller wasn't just a sign that I'd enjoy my visits or would keep coming back. It was also a sign that my therapy might actually work.

I'm sitting on my couch in my usual therapy uniform—sweatpants and a hoodie—ready to talk to Dr. Miller. I'm one of those people who feels much more relaxed with my contacts out, glasses on, and bra off. My brother always jokes that I can be counted on to wear a hoodie even if it's ninety degrees outside—and he's right. In therapy, I want to be as physically at ease as possible so I can be mentally present. Thursdays from 5:30 to 6:30 p.m. is the one hour a week that I have to focus on me—I call them "Therapy Thursdays." I'd love to have more time for myself, but I appreciate knowing that I at least have a nonnegotiable part of my week carved out. If I'm having a rough time at work, it's comforting to know there is always a protected space for me with someone who has my best interests at heart.

I open my appointment link, close all my other tabs—email,

Google, X—and put my phone in another room so I don't get distracted. I'm prepared to focus exclusively on my conversation with Dr. Miller.

Even though I really like and trust Dr. Miller, for some reason I'm always anxious right before we start. Often, this feeling is a sign of resistance, indicating there may be something I don't want to tell her or something I'm afraid she'll find out. Maybe that's true, even if I don't consciously know it. Or, maybe just letting myself be vulnerable makes me anxious. With vulnerability comes possible rejection; and in medicine, any vulnerability is seen as a weakness. Perhaps *anxious* isn't even a strong enough word to describe how I feel when sharing my innermost thoughts and feelings.

The computer makes a ringing sound, announcing that Dr. Miller has joined the "room," and I'm instantly comforted by the sight of her face on my screen. I let out an audible exhale.

Dr. Miller smiles and says hi, her straight, reddish brown hair falling down past her shoulders, her blue eyes looking, through her glasses, at my very dark brown ones. She is wearing a soft-looking blue sweater with the word *kindness* printed just below the neckline. I stifle an impulse to tell her I like it. *Me first*, I say in my head.

"So, where do you want to start?"

She initiates every appointment with this question, so I know what to expect. Many therapists structure their sessions with the same beginning and ending statements to help create a predictable and safe space, along with always starting and ending on time. It's a concept called "the frame," and keeping the frame can help foster trust. Even though I recognize exactly what she's doing, it works for me. Knowing how every visit will begin is not only comforting but also an easy, open-ended question I can take wherever I want.

I immediately launch into a tirade about my work week. Like so many of my patients, I always find it easier to start with fact recalls than with feelings, and mention present stressors rather than past ones. "Well, this week's been exhausting. I've been full patient-wise and haven't had a lot of breaks. And it seems like patients are really struggling, and then I'm struggling to help them with their struggling. Wow, I just said 'struggling' a lot, but it's all kinda meta." I smile, and so does she.

"Plus, I'm really starting to *hate* telehealth. I feel like it hurts my eyes by the end of the day, and sometimes even gives me a migraine. I just feel constantly distracted and even disconnected in some way. I don't know what that's about. I just can't stand it. . . ."

Dr. Miller interjects. "I'm just going to point out that I'm seeing you virtually, and if you don't like your work over a computer . . ."

"Ha!" I smile. "That's true . . . but this is different, I swear. I'd prefer to see you in person, *obviously*, but I can't, so I will see you however I can see you."

I don't say it to her, but I start thinking about how glad I am that we initially met in person. I think our bond is stronger for it. I'm not exactly sure why, but I feel the same way about my own patients. The screen creates some kind of barrier to connection, at least for me. Emerging data comparing face-to-face treatment with that conducted online shows significantly better scores in the creation of therapeutic alliances done in person.[2] At least my senses seem to line up with the research.

I continue going on about my week. At about minute eight, I start telling her about Megan and how much I've been thinking about our conversation since her visit a few days earlier.

"What about it stuck with you?" she asks.

"Well, I've always assumed I was a different kind of doctor than a Megan. That I somehow survived the hierarchy and my training with my emotions and empathy intact. But I think maybe I'm wrong."

"What makes you say that?"

"When I stop to think about it, a lot of what she was saying about her own emotions feels true for me, too. I remember, in medical school, receiving what were basically subjective evaluations of my personality, in which my supervisors said things like I 'made faces' and 'didn't take my job seriously' when I acted like myself around patients and supervisors, cracking a joke to a patient or laughing when a patient said one to me. When I learned all the nurses' names, my attendings said I was 'too cordial to nursing.' Like, they actually wrote that down about me. I remember wishing I could laugh and blow it off, and just be myself anyway, but instead I cried. Especially when I read the sentence on one evaluation: 'She needs to be reminded of her role in the hospital.'"

Dr. Miller purses her lips and I feel validated that this was, in fact, a very harsh thing to write. "Even though I know it's not healthy, that's still how things work in our system, which means the attendings won and I lost. I remember trying to work extra hours and come in early, hoping my work ethic would outweigh what they didn't like about me. But deep down, I knew that wasn't enough. I decided I had to hide myself and my personality. Before I said anything out loud to anyone, I would pause and ask myself what reaction I might provoke. That's a really hard thing for me to do, now and always, because I don't tend to have a great filter from my brain to my mouth. Still I tried, because I thought my evaluations might negatively affect my residency applications."

I pause to catch my breath. I can feel my muscles tightening just remembering the experience. Dr. Miller is just attentively listening.

"Talking to Megan, I'm realizing that what I thought was a subtle, temporary change in my behavior ended up being a bigger, more permanent one."

"What do you mean by that?" Dr. Miller asks, looking curious.

"I don't know. Maybe I'm dead inside."

"You're definitely not dead inside."

"Well, I'm for sure a product of medicine more than I realized. A week or so ago, I had a patient come in for an urgent appointment because his wife had died of COVID. We had been messaging back and forth, and I was treating him for his insomnia while she was in the hospital. The medication was helping him sleep, and his wife also seemed to be getting better. I felt like I was helping. He had even sent me her scans to show me that she was improving. And then, all of a sudden, she wasn't. I woke up to a message that she had died, and I asked the office to get him in that day if he could make it."

Dr. Miller listens intently, mostly nodding along.

"We ended up having a virtual appointment, and I was worried I wouldn't make it through the visit without crying. At one point, he was talking about his kids—they had three of them under the age of ten—and I could feel my eyes well up as my brain kept repeating *Stop! Don't you dare cry! You can't cry.* And my brain won. I actually stopped myself from crying."

"Stopped yourself?"

"Yes! He didn't notice a thing! And I was so proud of that. I thought, *Good job, Jessi. You didn't let even one tear fall in front of him.*"

Without skipping a beat or changing her expression, Dr. Miller responded: "And . . . why is that a good thing?"

"I don't know! That's the thing! I didn't think anything of it, until I was reflecting on my appointment with Megan. It's funny how that happens, but I honestly didn't really know what my own beliefs were about emotions in patient encounters. Then, suddenly, it all clicked and I sat up in bed last night and thought, *Whoa. That's fucked up.*"

"What's fucked up?" Dr. Miller asked, making me smile, because I love when she uses curse words. It feels a little like when your mom or your teacher does it—always surprising and a little cool.

"That I believe I'm not allowed to cry. That's what I was taught would make a good doctor. I can still hear the group of nurses who once told me in residency when I cried in front of them that *they'd never seen a doctor cry before.* And, in my shame and embarrassment, I took that to mean that doctors don't cry, at least the good ones. The ones who become chief residents. Even in the most authentic, human, and vulnerable moments with patients, that belief still wins out. It's like . . . I need to find ways to hide it, stop it, or deal with it, or maybe get out of medicine."

"What is 'it'?" she presses, kindly.

"Feeling? To stay in medicine, I feel like I need to stop my feelings." I pause briefly, eyes open. "*Wow. I see what you did there.*" This is one of those times I feel grateful that Dr. Miller is my therapist—when she leads me to an unexpected Aha! moment that even my own training hasn't allowed me to suss out.

She allows herself a satisfied smile as I compliment her therapy skills. "Thanks! But I know from doing this work myself, which is different from what you do but similar enough, that stopping feelings just isn't possible, at least in the long term." I nod, feeling heard. "What happens if you don't stop your feelings and you just let yourself feel?"

You mean like I keep telling my patients to do, but can't do myself? I think. Out loud, I say, "Truthfully? I hate even thinking about that."

"Why? What about it is so uncomfortable?"

"All of it, honestly. Big feelings get in the way of doing what I need to do to be successful. Especially the bad feelings."

"There aren't good or bad feelings, just feelings. The judgment doesn't need to be there."

"I know. But it is. Because, because . . . I worry what people will think of me."

Dr. Miller looks at me silently, likely hoping I'll keep talking.

"I worry people will think I'm too much. Too angry. Too emotional. Too sad. And that it will change their opinion of me."

The fear of being too much for people, especially when it comes to expressing emotions, is something I've always struggled with. It's part of why I didn't love being labeled "the emotional one" in my family.

I share this characteristic with so many of my patients, especially the female-identifying ones. Many women feel they have to hide their emotions, hide their human side, especially at work. It's hard enough for women to attain leadership roles; we can't have people thinking we're emotionally unstable, too.

It's something that a lot of women—and men, too—learn when

we are younger. Maybe we're crying about something on the play-ground, and people tell us not to cry because we're being a baby or weak. They might say, "You're fine, it's okay," and think they are being supportive, but really they're being invalidating because they're im-plying that we should suck it up and stop feeling. Because, after all, *It's okay. It's fine.*

Dr. Miller prods me carefully. "How do you think showing your emotions will change others' opinion of you?"

Because I trust her completely, I tell her the truth. "I project a cu-rated image of myself, especially at work, as someone who is compe-tent, hardworking, and caring at the same time. Having *big*, messy emotions runs counter to that image. It always has, since I was little."

She nods, then changes tack, slightly. "Have you ever had one of your doctors cry with you?" I think for a second, then shake my head *no*. She continues: "I can tell you that the one time my doctor cried with me—it was my own therapist actually—it was one of the best sessions I've ever had. Once I saw how I felt when she cried with me, I knew I didn't have to hide my own stories and feelings so much with my clients. I don't cry all the time, but I don't fight it if it comes."

"Oh, wow. Really, thanks for sharing that. That makes a lot of sense," I reply, grateful for her judicious use of self-disclosure and mentally filing it away for use with patients in the future. Another plus of being a psychiatrist in therapy—picking up tips from a good therapist. Especially tips they don't teach you, even discourage you from, in training.

But something in me is still resisting our conversation and where it's leading. "I'm . . . just not sure I can do it. I think, deep down, I'm still sensitive like my parents always said I was, but there are too many competing interests for me to let that out now."

Dr. Miller takes a deep breath. "It's hard, absolutely. But it isn't necessarily about showing your feelings all the time. It's more about caring about and noticing your feelings. I see that a lot when you're talking, and telling me about your patients, or about the struggles your friends and family are having. Even when you're asking me about me, it's different from when other patients just ask how I'm doing casually; you really care. But then, you spend a lot of time talking and worrying about other people's emotions, and not a lot of time on yours."

I think about the metaphor of putting on your own oxygen mask first before helping others, and then I vividly picture myself choking for air. I worry what Dr. Miller will think if I share that image—that I'm so clichéd, or as the kids say "basic," so I don't. There are still times I censor myself in our sessions. For instance, I haven't told her about all the negative thoughts in my head or about some of my more painful friendships ending. At least not yet. I can only be *so* vulnerable.

"Seriously, you—and your feelings—just need a seat at the table. You can start by asking yourself throughout the day how you're feeling, and pausing to note the answer. When is the last time you did that?"

"Is 'never' a possible answer?"

She smiles and I laugh awkwardly.

"What do you think about trying it?"

"Now?"

"Well, I meant at home, this week, but sure, what about now? How are you feeling?"

I fight the urge to say "fine."

"Appreciative."

7

"I'M OVER THIS shit, honestly . . . oops! Sorry . . . can I curse in here?"

I smile. "Of course you can. It's an emotional response, isn't it?"

My new patient Janet is a visibly pregnant woman with mid-shoulder-length, straight, dark hair who grins at me through the screen. "Yeah, I'm sorry, I don't mean over *you*, or having to be here really. I'm just over *all* of it. This whole being a nurse in a pandemic thing is truly as shitty as it gets."

"Oh, I knew what you meant. Don't worry, I had a feeling it was because of"—I gesture with my arms out wide— "all of this." I can only imagine what it's like to be a nurse right now.

What I know about Janet at this point can be boiled down to the few paragraphs of notes from her OB-GYN. She is a Filipina nurse in a local hospital, and eight months pregnant with her second child; her first, a daughter, is six years old. She's just shy of thirty years old, married, and has a history of postpartum depression.

Her gynecologist is the one who referred Janet to me, and who initially prescribed her antidepressant. I suspect her doctor worried that Janet's depression was worsening and wanted to make sure she was supported by a psychiatrist. And the fact that she's here now suggests to me that *something* must have changed in her life.

I point those things out as I try to get more information in my typical first-visit way. "So, I know you have a history of depression and are on a medication. I can see your chart from your OB. . . . But

74

still, it's always better to hear what's going on directly from you. So, tell me what brings you to me today?"

Janet leans into the screen and says, "Well, I was doing alright with the pregnancy and my mood, and feeling good on the Zoloft, which I started after my first pregnancy. It's the only medication I've ever been on. But then our hospital really started to fill up with COVID patients and . . . it's just been . . . honestly we don't know what to do for the patients and we have nowhere to put them. It's a lot."

I notice Janet talks with her hands. I appreciate that, because otherwise I can really only see, well, *read,* her face on the screen. "We converted the recovery rooms from surgeries into COVID rooms, and we still need more beds. And to add insult to injury, this week was my second week having to work in the ICU instead of oncology, where I've worked as a nurse since I got out of school. They call it 're-deployment'—like we're soldiers or something."

I visibly cringe. "To be honest, I struggle some with those war analogies, too—like *redeployed, frontline,*" I admit. "I feel like it's a way to act like we're in wartime, but we aren't in a war."

I catch myself thinking about how, unlike Janet, I'm behind my computer, safe and away from COVID patients, while she's in the ICU every day, at risk and pregnant. I feel instantly overwhelmed by guilt, so I start talking, hoping that turning my focus back to her will make the guilt go away. "I don't know what it's like to change fields at any time, let alone during a pandemic, but I can guess. You're not the only patient of mine who has mentioned having to do that." I notice that I've raised my voice by the time I get to the end of my sentence.

I feel angry, and though I don't say this to her, I think my anger is only slightly about her experience; it's more grounded in an email I received from our hospital yesterday. The message went out to all clinical providers, and included a survey asking about our medical and ICU skills, presumably in case they need us to work somewhere else. In processing the survey, I had long text-message discussions with friends about the concept of redeployment. I feel strongly that redeploying is not really a reasonable expectation for people who have trained for years to specialize in a field of medicine, like psychiatry, until we feel that's all we can do (which is probably the truth). Beyond something like an in-flight emergency, no one ever told us in training that we could suddenly be directed to practice whatever other field we happened to be needed for, whether it's the ER or ICU. To me, this new development makes me feel as if I'm a pawn in the system, instead of an expert in something specific. But any time I try to say something like "I'm not sure I would even agree to do it," many of my friends act as if I've said something sacrilegious. So, I have learned to keep my thoughts and feelings to myself, as I have had to do with so many conversations before.

My opinions aside, I have never worked a single day in the ICU. That choice was deliberate. Emotionally, I realized that I'm not cut out for it, and since I didn't have to do it to become a psychiatrist, I chose not to. One of the reasons I picked psychiatry is that my personality is a good fit for the field. Having to switch to a field characterized by chronic urgency and a lot of exposure to death would very likely affect me mentally, and not in a good way. That awareness helps me empathize with patients like Janet, who are being forced to switch. It also makes me really anxious about the what-ifs.

Janet responds by thanking me for understanding, adding, "I bet a lot of people are struggling with this situation, but we mostly don't talk about any of it in healthcare. Honestly, when they first asked me to work in the ICU, I was happy to do it. I felt like I'd been called to action to help." She looks down, letting out another long sigh. "But it's not what I thought it'd be. Plus, I miss oncology."

"Can you tell me more about that?" I ask gently, hoping to begin to pry open what is likely a huge can of worms.

"Well, my whole job is different now. I work longer hours, and if it's any sign of how much more I'm running around, I'm getting something like 15,000 steps a day, according to my fitness watch. Obviously, I'm also doing a different kind of nursing, and it's not like anything I've ever experienced before. All I hear all day are codes—the beeps of the machines, the hustle of people trying to save a life, the pagers going off in the distance . . ."

She trails off as if the sounds are conjuring up a memory she is not yet ready to share. I think about how much I hate the sound of my pager, and how it instantly brings up every stressful and negative experience I've had on call. I wonder what she's thinking, but maybe she has not even had the time to stop and think. I don't call it out and into actual awareness, like I might in a later appointment. She does not know or trust me yet. I don't want her to shut down and shut me out.

"Codes just happen, over and over," she continues. "We can't get people help fast enough. Like, I'm in the middle of helping someone get intubated, and there is a code down the hall. The whole experience is chaotic and stressful. Sometimes, it doesn't even seem real."

"Thank you for sharing all of that with me," I start with, hoping to validate all that she has already told me and acknowledge that reliving it must not be easy. At the same time, hearing all this is emotional and heavy for me. To protect myself, I've mostly removed myself from my body and my feelings as she speaks—something I learned to do in training when I was first bombarded with patients' traumatic stories. It's like I'm an observer, rather than actually being there, and if I'm not really there, the conversation and triggers can't hurt me. It's a form of dissociation—disconnecting from one's feelings, thoughts, memories, or identity. For me, it isn't exactly conscious, but it does involve my stepping away from the visit with a patient explaining their trauma, and detaching from myself. It's subtle and a patient wouldn't notice; I am there physically, though not emotionally. Often, it's a necessary move for an empath who could easily feel flooded and affected by the end of a day with patients and their stories. I'm good at it, which helps in the moment, but it is also another reason why I have trouble identifying my own feelings, as Dr. Miller has noticed. Somehow I have no problem identifying them in others.

"Here is something I wonder. I'm not a nurse, so maybe I just don't know, but when you think about working on oncology, and then are working now in the ICU, how is it different? Like, I could be super-ignorant, but I'd guess you have seen really sick patients and a lot of death before, right?" I ask not for my own education or under-standing but, rather, because the way Janet perceives this difference is key for me in understanding her psychological reactions to what she is going through now.

"Well, yes, I saw sick patients all the time in oncology, but the *way* in which COVID patients are sick is something I've never seen before. It really takes me outside my comfort zone. I feel like a new grad right out of nursing school, or something. I'll walk into a room to see a patient, and I don't know what to expect or what's going to happen. Patients you don't think are going to code end up coding, and patients you thought were going to code don't. It just doesn't seem to make any sense, and I feel out of control. My years of nurs-ing haven't prepared me for this. And the hospital sure as shit hasn't, either."

"What do you mean by that?" I ask, aware that I'm starting a con-versation that almost every healthcare worker I have ever met has *strong* opinions about.

"Well, it normally takes months of training to change fields to work as an ICU nurse, with classes and supervision on the floor. But they gave us *one week* of prep, with links to webinars and a twenty-page take-home packet."

"One week?" I echo, to encourage her to continue speaking but also, mostly, because I'm stunned.

"Yes. One week. That's all. Like I can just up and become an ICU nurse in one week, in a fucking pandemic. . . . Ha! Saying it out loud, it just sounds so ridiculous."

It does, but it's not an anomaly. A study of healthcare workers in the UK[1] during the pandemic found that very few were adequately trained for their redeployment and their skills were often not consid-ered before they were sent to different units to work. And because hospitals did not (or could not) match the skills of the staff to the skills needed in the new work areas, they often created more problems than they solved.

Janet pauses again and then continues, "And, it's just been one thing after another. I don't know how to do some of the important stuff on the unit, like managing oxygen and medications I've never used before, like particular sedatives. I was literally asking Siri, 'Hey Siri, How do you manage a ventilator?' I feel incompetent and worried that someone will find me out. Not my colleagues, because they're all in the same boat, but families or patients. I feel like it's Halloween and I'm wearing the costume of an ICU nurse."

"That all seems so disconcerting," I tell her, "but it does sound like you're doing what you can do. Of course, you're also pregnant, so I'd imagine that makes things more . . . complicated."

She nods. "Complicated is an understatement. I'm like a guinea pig. Since the start of the pandemic, no one has known what to do, period, but especially with pregnant people. At the very beginning of the pandemic, I was freaking out about my exposure and kept asking my OB, 'What do you think about me working through this? Is this a good idea?' Not only did she not know, but she didn't want to risk guessing and being wrong. Or, be too cautious and tell me—and all her pregnant healthcare-worker patients—that we couldn't work during a tremendous staff shortage. So, instead, she didn't tell me anything. She just hemmed and hawed and said, 'We don't know.' No one knew. But I had a gut feeling that COVID *had* to be worse in pregnancy."

"What do you think that gut feeling was about?"

"Well, anxiety or fear seems about right. But I was talking to my best work friend, a male nurse, and he helped me figure it out. He said bluntly, 'Pregnant women are a *niiiiiightmare* to intubate. They require a ridiculous amount of meds, and you know, their physiology is different. That's why you don't want to get COVID, silly.' And it clicked. It was one of those times when having medical knowledge makes things worse, not better. I was worried I would get COVID, and that if I did, I would be harder to care for because of my pregnancy, or maybe I'd need to be intubated and the only person who was around to do that was someone who had been redeployed, like me, and wouldn't know how. I've basically just resigned myself to the fact that if I get sick, I will die. And . . . that's terrifying."

I asked her if her co-workers had been protective of her, and if she had experienced that culture of caring that typically leads people to give up their seat on a crowded train or bus.

Janet replied, "I expected that, because that was how it was when I was pregnant with Maddy, my first kid. Everyone was more compassionate. But now, because everybody is going through the pandemic and scared for themselves and their families, it's different. Like that little bit of extra something you get when you're pregnant, that little extra concern you get from co-workers—it's gone." I don't say this out loud, but I wonder if this, for lack of a better word, selfishness, has to do with everyone being so concerned for their own physiologic needs; it makes sense that people aren't helping others as much. They can barely help themselves.

"I never thought about that," I say. But now, of course, I'm going to ask my friends who are pregnant if it has been the same for them, while also trying to do better and find ways to still care for them extra. "But, it makes sense why all of that might make your mood worse right now. I wonder, too, if aside from pregnancy, you have any added triggers or pressure from being a mom to Maddy. . . ."

My talking points are now coming straight from conversations with the doctor-moms in my life—my best friend from residency, my sister, and my sister-in-law. But I don't tell Janet that because it isn't about me or my family.

"Oh gosh, yes. I mean, Maddy is in kindergarten, but they aren't meeting in person and virtual is only effective for, like, five minutes with a kid her age, so I end up having to really help when I'm home."

"With all of your free time," I add, sarcastically.

Janet replies, with equivalent sarcasm, "Oh, yes, *all* of my free time. It's *soooo* easy. And so are the times when I read the news or watch TV and I start to cry, and Maddy says, 'Mommy, Mommy, what's wrong?' I try to answer in a way she'll understand, but I must be saying something wrong, because now she gets really worried about me when I go into work; she knows that's where the virus is. As if going to work where the virus is wasn't hard enough for me already."

I think people forget that many of the healthcare workers showing up to work in the pandemic are parents, too, experiencing all the stressors of the healthcare environment, plus everything that comes with parenthood, or pregnancy, or both. From what I see with friends who are pregnant or have just given birth, COVID seems to heighten the stress of being a new mother times about a thousand percent. That's the scientific number.

It's no wonder that studies done about pregnancy as the pandemic progressed have shown perceived threats to the life of the mother and baby were linked to higher symptoms of depression and anxiety.[2] Plus, once mothers gave birth, they were significantly more likely to experience postpartum anxiety and depression.[3] In fact, mothers were 2.6 times more likely to have postpartum depression during the pandemic than before.

Though not widely studied, female healthcare workers were also found to be especially vulnerable to these symptoms, further compounding existing gender inequities in medicine. In a cohort study of physicians conducted in August 2020,[4] physician mothers were more likely than physician fathers to be responsible for the schooling, childcare, and household tasks. They also experienced more depression and anxiety. Interestingly, the gender difference for depression among physician parents was not seen in patient samples before the pandemic.

To put it plainly, the pandemic just made everything worse, including underlying and existing gender disparities and stressors.

Switching topics, I ask Janet about PPE, and whether she has the protective gear that she needs at work.

"Well, I am *extremely* cautious, more so than anyone else, because I'm pregnant," she says.

"Even though everyone is wearing an N-95 at work, two or so months into this thing, I've been wearing one since the beginning, when everyone else was still wearing surgical masks. I also wore gloves and a face shield, and anything else I could find to protect me. At one point, a patient came in unresponsive, and because I wanted to wear all the gear, it took me much longer to get ready to help than anyone else. I was watching everyone staring at me, but I just kept thinking, *I am not risking myself and my baby . . . sorry, not sorry.* Still, I was honestly worried they would fire me for refusing to care for a patient or something."

"Did they say that to you?"

"No, but they weren't really supportive, either. They were giving me 'Suck it up and do your job and help people no matter what, you're a nurse, you signed up for this' kind of stares."

"But, should you? Suck it up and do your job?"

"I have been, but I'm conflicted, which is why my heart is constantly going like 120 beats per minute."

"What do you think that's telling you? Your heartbeat, I mean." I say this because thanks, in part, to Bessel van der Kolk, somewhat controversial psychiatrist and author, we know the body keeps the score (from his book with the same title), and it's always trying to tell us something. Even if we do not consciously remember a difficult event or a trauma or feel emotionally triggered by it, our bodies sometimes still warn us and sound the alarm (increasing our heart rate, for example).

She pauses as if to listen to her heartbeat and then replies, "That I'm not comfortable, or safe. Everything is so different from what we were always told. Like, we learned masks were single use and then all of the sudden we're using them for days, weeks even, and are told that it's fine. Why should we trust that?"

"It can definitely feel like the people making the rules—the administration—are not on your side," I acknowledge. "And that what you are being asked to do is against your morals, and everything you learned to be right and safe."

"Yes, exactly that."

I use the word *morals* with Janet intentionally. For nurses,[5] in particular, the pandemic compounded existing moral strains. There is a term—*moral injury*—that refers to the overall impact of participating in, failing to prevent, or even witnessing acts that go against your moral beliefs.[6] The term is a military one, like *redeployment*, and it refers to having healthcare workers do things that go against what they know is right—for themselves and for their patients. Like most things, the pandemic didn't create moral injury in medicine, but it created an environment ripe for more of it.

Moral injury doesn't just cause an in-the-moment strain. It can potentially lead to long-lasting mental health outcomes, like depression, PTSD, substance use, and suicidal thoughts.[7] One way to prevent that from happening is to talk about decision-making in groups, out loud.[8] Validation from others that you made the right or only possible decision can help people get through with less moral injury. Ideally, those discussions would happen in real time. When they don't, and they often don't (or aren't allowed by leadership), my job is to lend an ear in a system that isn't ready to talk about all this yet.

"Honestly, it feels like the people in charge are getting bonuses while I'm going to work every day, pregnant, and in harm's way," Janet continues. "I know so many co-workers and friends across the country who are writing out their wills and telling their kids their wishes."

"I have had friends and family do that, too. It's the right thing to do, I guess, but it brings death that much closer."

"Yes, exactly! But, you don't see the CEOs doing that from their islands in the Caribbean." She lets out a sarcastic laugh and I do, too.

"The system plays such a big role in people's mental health, and yet it doesn't change much," Janet says, echoing my feelings exactly. "They think telling healthcare workers 'Thank you' with a banner as we enter the hospital or that throwing us a pizza party will help."

Somehow in unison we both say, "It won't."

I then add, "I hate to switch gears, but we are almost out of time today, and I wanted to make sure I addressed the reason you are here with me, and to check in about medication."

"It's okay, I get it."

"So, it doesn't sound to me like you are actively depressed—a little anxious maybe, frustrated and irritable, too, which could be related, I guess—but all that seems grounded in valid experiences and seems like your medication is helping in some capacity. Do you feel depressed?"

"It's possible some of that is there still, but I still have joy in things, and it's not like I'm sad. I also feel like so much of it is situational. As you point out, work, pregnancy, teaching my kid at home—there are a lot of situations that lead me to say, 'That's why I feel this way.'"

"I get that, I do. But keeping in mind that a lot of those stressors aren't going to change tomorrow, do you feel like they are interfering in your daily life—enough that you want to change meds or your dose?"

"After talking it all out just now, if it's okay with you I'd really like to not mess with medication while I'm pregnant. I feel okay . . . enough . . . and even though I know there is low risk to the baby, which is why I decided to stay on meds in the first place, I'd rather not add *more*. I would love to keep things as they are right now." She points out that maybe she would start therapy or mindfulness as a practice again, but that she really wants to stay connected to me, just in case. "I just don't know that I will be okay when the baby is actually out in the world, so it feels a bit safer knowing you're here."

"Of course! I totally understand, and that's a common reaction to medications in pregnancy. Just know that you can always change your mind. Depression and anxiety themselves have their own risks to the baby that are also worth weighing." She nods and I emphasize, "I'm not going anywhere. I'm here, whenever."

"Winter, spring, summer, or fall . . ."

"Yep. All you have to do is call."

We both laugh a little at my extreme cheesiness. There's not much else we can do.

8

THIS MORNING, I open the fridge and, right next to the nonfat milk and eggs, is a carton of ice cream from the night before, soft and melting. I'd normally laugh about my absentmindedness and not read into it, but given my homework assignment from my last therapy session—*Ask yourself how you are doing*—it seems like a huge red flag.

Like many of my patients, I'm bad at doing therapy homework. My therapist knows this, but she still slips in suggestions for things for me to try every once in a while. The evidence of my failures is subtle, but if you look closely you will see at my bedside half-read books she has suggested (like one on self-compassion, by Kristin Neff). There's also a downloaded CALM app on my phone for bedtime stories and a never-plugged-in alarm clock from the time she suggested I try moving my phone away from my bedside.

With the melted ice cream, it's like the universe is reminding me I haven't checked on myself or my feelings at all—or my supposedly frozen desserts. I think, *Psychiatrist mood check: How are you feeling?*

The truth is, I'm not doing very well at all.

For one thing, I don't sleep much. Lately, I've been staying up until 2 or 3 in the morning, "doomscrolling" posts on social media from healthcare workers all over the country. On each one, I click Like, or add a comment about how what they're doing matters and that they are allowed to have whatever feelings they need to have about it. If only I listened to myself.

I have this urge to be supportive and validating of their struggles because I'm afraid no one else will be. I've taken it upon myself almost as if it's a job, and I can't seem to stop. I can't seem to let go. I think, *If I sleep, someone might not be there for them*, as if I have more hours or energy to give. In addition to my online "patients" and my ever-increasing real ones, I've been giving four or five weekly mental health talks around the hospital, a routine I fondly refer to as my "trade show." I speak for anywhere from ten to forty-five minutes, and I focus on making sure that everyone, from business administrators to anesthesiologists, knows all about our department's mental health resources. Yet the department has been on overdrive since the pandemic started. We added a support phone line that the psychiatry department is staffing on-call, we started drop-in mental health skills and support groups, and we greatly expanded our outpatient therapy and psychiatry treatment options for healthcare workers and their families, with the goal of getting them in for their first appointment within two weeks.

When the pandemic started, it was clear to me that things wouldn't be good for healthcare workers in terms of their mental health. It wasn't great before, and the pandemic, I suspected, would make things worse. Which is why I emailed the head of our department and asked, almost nonchalantly, "What are we planning to do for the mental health of our own people?" To which he replied, "I don't know, Jessi, what are we going to do?"

Before I knew it, a few of my peers and I were designing the psychiatry department's role and response to support the university system during COVID. Like my patient Janet, I felt called to help, felt like I *needed* to help. Only, I didn't realize how much extra work that would be—measured not just in terms of hours but also in emotions. Dr. Miller keeps telling me that my talks don't cover fun or uplifting topics, and that takes a toll. Every Friday evening, as I collapse onto my couch and don't wake up until noon on Saturday, I realize just how right she is.

I sigh and try to distract myself from some uncomfortable feelings by thinking about how at least I did complete my assignment. I make a mental note to tell Dr. Miller so I can get a gold star. After all, I never did outgrow my need for positive reinforcement.

My thoughts, however, are somehow fixated on the word *struggling* and as it repeats in my head, my neck starts to tense up and I feel my heart beating faster. I don't like the feeling, so I decide to make it go away. Extrovert that I am, my go-to coping move used to be reaching out to a friend; before the pandemic, it felt I had that option in spades. My friends represent every stage of my life and are scattered all over the country, whether they are people I once went to school with, as far back as elementary school, or they are those I have worked with. Some I have met in random ways, a specialty of mine; for example, the photographers I clicked with when I was a bridesmaid in a friend's wedding; the news reporter who interviewed me once; the friend my former OB-GYN excitedly introduced me to when she found out I was moving to her city; or the vet who had unexpectedly to euthanize my last dog. I'm always on the lookout for people I can connect with, because I always need to be doing things, and the more people I can do them with, the better. Being a good friend is also a core value of mine.

It's different now, though. I can't just make new friends, or even make a plan to look forward to. I can't go down my list of usual suspects and find someone who is free to do something . . . because there is nothing to be free for. There are no concerts, movies, or comedy shows—my favorite activities—and certainly there are no vacations. Everyone else is focused on themselves and their families, and I can't blame them.

I look down at my phone and think about texting a friend in California, but I stop myself. It's only 6 a.m. there. Also, I don't know what I would say to her, other than "Hi, I miss humans."

I guess this is what loneliness feels like. I've lived alone for a long time, but oddly I've never truly felt lonely before. That may sound strange for a single woman in her thirties, but I've always had friends, or family, or colleagues, or even my patients around—so much so that I don't tend to pine for a partner. The loneliness I feel isn't for a romantic relationship; I'm not eating my melted ice cream from the carton, belting out "All by Myself" à la Bridget Jones. What I feel is a longing for the life I was enjoying before the pandemic and the energy that being around people gave me.

With all that gone now, I feel depleted. Video calls with friends, even virtual trivia games or movie nights, just don't fill me up the same way, though these distractions are better than nothing. When no one is on the screen, it's quiet, and I don't like the quiet. The same way I push down big feelings and fight silence in my therapy sessions, I go to great lengths to avoid it at home, even if I don't always know I'm doing that.

"I've been writing a lot," I tell Dr. Miller at the start of my next appointment.

"I've noticed."

I smile, knowing that if she is saying that, she has seen my name pop up somewhere in an article I've written or a story I've been interviewed for. I like the fact that she has clearly thought about me outside of our appointments—the dream of most patients. People want to be liked in general, but there is a specific kind of desire to be liked by one's therapist. As a therapist myself, I'd love to say we don't have favorites, but I know I do, which means Dr. Miller probably does, too. I don't treat patients any differently, but I feel different with them— happier maybe? With Dr. Miller, I try to be subtle about my delight that she has noticed my outside-of-session activities, so as not to seem creepy. In my mind, though, I'm wondering if I'm a favorite.

She continues, "Does it seem like you're doing more than usual?"

I pause to think. "Yeah, I mean I did something like twelve things besides work this past month," I admit. When I say "things besides work," I mean that in my "free time" I've written articles and op-eds, have given talks all over the country (on Zoom), and have appeared as an expert in all kinds of media, usually talking about burnout and coping skills during COVID. Even though Dr. Miller hasn't said anything judgmental, I feel a bit defensive. "There's a lot of stuff to write and talk about right now," I explain. "Our mental health is . . . not . . . great, especially in the populations I treat." I look at Dr. Miller to see if her facial expression has changed. It hasn't.

I continue, "But a friend of mine noticed everything I was doing and asked me if something was wrong. Like my sheer output was a sign of my mental state."

"That was perceptive of her. What do you make of that?"

I laugh. "I mean, most of my friends are perceptive for a living, so I guess I have that, for better or worse. Still, I felt a bit criticized. I wanted to tell her, 'I'm writing articles because there is something to write about!' Kind of like what I just said to you. I didn't say it, even though I think it's true. But I guess it may also be something I'm telling myself—to rationalize."

I shift positions on the couch and take a sip of water. Suddenly I feel uncomfortable. I'm sure Dr. Miller sees this and will read into it, but she only asks me to clarify what I mean, which is a relief.

"Well, when I take on writing assignments or agree to give a talk, I can basically be busy all the time. It fills in the pauses, so I don't have to be by myself or have time to think about how I'm by myself."

Another pause. "And . . . if you did think about that?"

"I think I'd be overwhelmed with sad feelings and I'd have to admit that this pandemic is affecting me, too."

"Would that be horrible to say out loud?"

"I just . . . well, of course it *is* affecting me. But I feel guilty saying that from behind my computer, childless, while I listen to all the stuff my patients in healthcare and those with little kids are dealing with."

"I can see why you would think that, but you have to be careful comparing yourself to your patients. You can usually never win that battle."

She's right. I think about all I've heard from my patients today alone, and how much hurt is in the world right now. I also consider how so many of my patients think they don't deserve to feel bad because their problems are *just* work related. "But I'm not dying" is also a common thing they say. I recognize I'm doing the same thing.

There's a term for a lot of the patients I see—*high functioning*—which basically means that they are continuing to work or go to school, with an implied judgment that if they can do that, maybe their problems aren't so bad. I know from what I'm hearing that that often isn't the case, that even though they're "functioning," they're often smiling through the pain. Which is why I feel driven to do all that I'm doing to help them. Most people would have described me that way in the past, too.

"I think I just feel better when I *do* things," I tell Dr. Miller, "especially when those things are advocacy related and help people. That's why I'm so active on social media and doing so much extra at work. I just want to help however I can. I want to make myself essential."

Dr. Miller interjects, "That goal—of being essential—is important for you to have named out loud." *Thanks,* I think. *Too bad noticing it doesn't make me feel better.* Honestly, ever since they told me I was nonessential, I've had a chip on my shoulder about it. It's hard to be so busy and work so hard, and at the same time be told that the work I do, and by extension mental health in general, isn't considered essential by others. It's disorienting.

"I also wonder," she continues, "if it's more than just that working hard makes you feel better because you're helping people, that it's also that the structure of work, the achievement and feedback you get from work, actually helps you, too."

I shift on the couch again and really pause to think before I ask my next question, which comes to me like an epiphany. "Can work be . . . a coping skill?"

Dr. Miller smiles. "Well, yes, I think so. Do you think you use it like that?"

"Well, now I do! I never thought about it before, but I do think I'm saying yes to more things right now because I have nowhere else to be, no friends to see. A lot of feelings to hide. It works, too, except for the times when I look at my schedule, get angry, and wonder, *Why am I so busy?* And then realize I did it to myself."

"I know the feeling," Dr. Miller interjects with a smile.

"I'll try to notice it more. And earlier. And to also think about what's going on in my life or the world that is driving me to do and just keep doing."

Dr. Miller's eyes narrow as she adds, "And if I can be instructive, which I hate to be . . . "

"Seriously, tell me what to do . . ." I respond half-jokingly, but also somewhat seriously.

"Maybe also try to make work not the *only* thing you are doing to cope?"

I want to say absolutely, and get to it, but in reality I don't have hobbies. I'm not sure I ever have had any—other than pastimes related to work and achievement. As I hear myself explaining this to Dr. Miller, I sound so familiar. The no-hobbies thing is common among my healthcare-worker patients. When school takes up so much time and energy, it's hard to do much else, and then that's how you're set up as you move into your adult life: busy and focused. I used to play the piano and act in school plays, but I gave those things up for school and the swim team. And eventually I just landed on school.

Dr. Miller wants me to find things I enjoy again, but when I can't think of anything to do or try, she recommends I look at a "pleasant activities" list. That's a list of everything from bubble baths to running. It has good ideas for those of us who would otherwise take hours to even come up with choices for where to go out to dinner, if a friend didn't just go ahead and choose, or at least narrow down the options. The list is that friend, but for hobbies. I've given these lists to patients, but never looked at them for myself—probably because they seem so simple, silly even. Though maybe that's why they work.

She adds, "The world has gotten flipped upside down, and now you have to figure out what you can do, alone."

"You know what I realized?" She looks back at me, telling me to go on.

"I think you're my most consistent relationship right now."

9

THE NEXT PATIENT on my schedule today is Luke, the resident with new symptoms of OCD. I quickly look through his chart to remember what we talked about last time: his fear of infection and other symptoms related to the virus, and his pattern of repeating the number three. Also, my suggestion that he start exposure and response prevention (ERP) therapy (often called simply exposure therapy) and the list of possible medications he could take that I gave him to review. It's been close to three months since I last saw him; time is passing weirdly now, with minutes and hours going so slowly that it can be hard to keep track of the days of the week. And yet, weeks are also speeding by.

When I see Luke on my screen, I offhandedly ask, "How are you?"

I regret it immediately. For one, it's an overused question and not typically meant to evoke actual vulnerability. Most of us, when someone asks us this, don't have the time or energy for giving a real answer. Society is generally okay with that; we've decided it's polite, even acceptable to answer on autopilot. But it isn't to me. To help Luke as his psychiatrist, I need the real answer.

Predictably, he responds, "I'm fine." "Fine" is often a joke among mental health practitioners because it usually means the person, like me so many times, is anything *but* fine. We've even given it an acronym: Feelings I'm Not Expressing.

Luke then pauses briefly and asks, "How about you?"

This is the other issue with the how-are-you question: It begs to be reciprocated. But that's far removed from the purpose of our session. And in this kind of situation, we psychiatrists aren't *supposed* to talk about ourselves.

Still, I notice something about the quality of Luke's voice—something I've noticed in a lot of my patients lately. I can tell he's genuinely curious about my well-being, that he wants to know the truth. He won't be satisfied with the answer they teach us to give when we are in training, which is basically to ask why someone is asking about us in the first place, turning the question back on them.

I feel myself desperately wanting to tell Luke the truth, while ensuring him I'm safe and coping so he knows I can take good care of him. Psychologically speaking, I suspect this is the core reason for his question. I'm living through a pandemic, too, and he's worried about my ability to help him.

How am I? I think, trying to come up with an appropriate answer. The truth is that I'm busy and tired, but I don't yet know what deeper emotions those feelings are masking. I don't tell him that, though, because I worry he wouldn't trust a psychiatrist who can't figure out her own feelings. All that comes out of my mouth is "I'm hangin' in."

"I get that," he nods, and we have a moment when we look at each other through the screens with what feels like mutual respect for our different roles in healthcare at this moment in time, and how hard it's been. Something tells me he feels satisfied with my response, even though it wasn't long or heavy. It was enough to move us forward.

"So, what's been going on since I saw you last?" I ask, hoping to get a more detailed reply.

"Well, I know it's been a little while, but I've been going to the therapy you recommended and liking it. I think it's helping, though it's a slow improvement."

"Therapy is a bit tricky like that," I respond. "It takes time, and it can even feel as if your problems are getting worse before they get better. At the beginning, exposure therapy might cause much more anxiety and maybe it will even mess with your sleep. But after you do it a number of times, those things won't bother you as much, and eventually, hopefully, not at all."

Luke sits up a bit straighter. "Yeah, that's exactly how it's been! Right now, I'm working on handling the groceries delivered to my house. My therapist tells me that I can't immediately wipe the groceries down with bleach wipes, as much as my OCD makes me want to. First, I have to hold an item of my choice for a minute, which can still feel overwhelming sometimes. But luckily my therapist warned me about all of it before we started. I'm glad he did, or I would've been pissed off and thought it wasn't working."

"You're not alone in that!" I say. I start to think of all my patients who've mentioned feeling worse because of what they're working on in therapy, particularly the ones like Luke focusing on their exposures, and others who are doing trauma-focused therapy. So many of them even stop going because of it. "There's a saying in therapy," I tell Luke, "you have to go through it to get through it. And I think it's pretty spot on for a lot of people. It just takes time."

For my patients, this is one of the most surprising things about therapy—how long it can take to feel better. Most of us aren't used to confronting our issues head on, and when we do, we face not only our own resistance but also years of baggage to unpack. In a review of randomized controlled trials for OCD, the mean number of therapy sessions for a patient was 14.7, but that length can vary by symptom severity and other co-occurring diagnoses.[1] Given that employers usually cover only three to five sessions at a lowered rate or for free in their insurance plans, it is no wonder there are so many barriers to even starting treatment, as well as the high rates of drop-outs over time. Some conditions, like trauma or even burnout, might require longer time frames—something that therapy helps us work on as well. What I don't say to Luke is how I'm still learning to accept that myself with Dr. Miller, as I now cross over four years of weekly therapy.

"I wish I had more time," he says, looking defeated. "Time for anything outside of being a resident, honestly. But I had to go on temporary leave just to make it to therapy as often as my therapist wants me to go."

My heart flutters a bit in my chest, and I notice I feel a little sad for him for having to take a leave. As much as I thought it could happen, and maybe even should have happened earlier, I also wish I'd been wrong.

"How often are you going, now, to therapy?" I ask, trying to understand the "dose" of ERP his clinician has prescribed. The frequency is another factor that can help me understand the severity of Luke's symptoms. While it's true that someone doing therapy might need to go to more or longer sessions up front anyway, there's still a difference between advising someone to go more than once a week and someone who can get away with going monthly, biweekly, or even weekly.

"They started me with three times a week! Do you believe it?" Luke says, looking surprised himself.

I smile sympathetically, and as I'm pretty sure his question is rhetorical, I don't respond. Still, in my head I'm thinking that three times a week is definitely frequent.

"I was confused at first and repeatedly asked my therapist, 'Are you sure?'" Luke continues. "And when he explained why, I knew it was the right choice. I knew if I was ever going to get better that I needed to go that often, but I wish I could go to intensive therapy and still be a full-time resident, or even part time."

"That must've been a really hard decision for you to make— to take time off," I say quietly with sincere empathy and also with genuine concern for his mental well-being. "I know how much work means to you."

Because it means the same to me, I think. He looks down and away, almost as if he is going to tear up, but he doesn't. He just nods.

I wonder a lot about identity and medicine, and how much a

resident like Luke, who is still in training, has already been defined by his career. After all, he's gone through years of classes, spending time and money to get where he is right now, sacrificing friendships and relationships, and even vacations. I thought about dropping out of medical school at more than a few points along the way, and each time I decided I had already invested too much to simply stop. I couldn't imagine starting over or doing anything else. I wouldn't even know what that something else could be. That was also the message I got from almost everyone else I talked to about it. "How many people can even say they got into med school?" was a common refrain, as they encouraged me to just finish.

But pushing through to the end of his residency, even though he is so close to finishing, clearly isn't an option right now for Luke. Whatever he was hoping for, his body and mind have other plans. That makes me feel terrible for him, as I can see how much he wants it. The unknown of it all, including when or even if he might be well enough to return to work, must also be unbearable at times.

Speaking from the experiences of patients, friends, and myself, I add, "The medical field is also inherently set up to make you feel as if you're doing something wrong if you need to take time off, as if you're breaking a cardinal rule. Has it been like that for you?"

"Honestly?"

"Yes."

"It feels like I'm letting down my colleagues and patients at a time when everyone needs me most. It's as if I've gone AWOL and abandoned the troops during active war."

I try to hide my response to that painful war metaphor, seemingly a default analogy for what healthcare workers can't otherwise articulate, even if we all hate when others use it. But inside, I feel angry and sad at the same time. Which, come to think of it, is probably what he feels, too.

———————

Physicians are taught early on to go to work no matter what, even if they're sick. As my friends and colleagues like to say, the only way medical professionals are allowed to stay home sick is if they show up to work first and are then sent home. I've heard this called, from various people, "Turning up to prove you're dead." Often, as with Luke, it's because we don't want to burden our colleagues with more work or worry about letting patients down.[2]

Showing up to work sick is a concept known as *presenteeism*, and while it's not as easily measured as absenteeism, it's a common phenomenon and a costly one.[3] Workers across many industries fear being fired for missing a day on the job, or don't have paid sick days, so they show up when they're ill (a key reason for the rampant spread of COVID in some households). American culture also tends to value work over self-care. It's not surprising, then, that the symptoms of burnout—high emotional exhaustion and cynicism—are associated with more presenteeism.[4]

Yet in medicine, working while you're sick can also hurt or infect patients, some of whom might already be quite sick themselves. In one survey of physicians and advanced practice providers such as physician associates and nurse practitioners, nearly all agreed with the statement that working while sick puts patients at risk. Yet that belief didn't change their behavior. More than 83 percent noted that they'd worked while sick at least once in the prior year and more than 9 percent reported at least five times.[5] This remained true even when people were obviously contagious.[6] Even worse, more than half of the healthcare workers who care for immunocompromised transplant recipients—patients who literally cannot fight infection, meaning they can die from being exposed—admitted to working while being sick with flu-like symptoms.[7] I'm ashamed to admit that as a resident, I also worked when I was ill and coughing (with a mask!), even though I was around hospitalized patients. A nurse had to fight with my attending to send me home.

Despite the risk to ourselves and our patients, and how unacceptable we know it is to put patients at risk when we may be contagious, the cultural norm of showing up no matter what wins out in medicine, even if it isn't healthy for anyone. And that's the expectation for people with *physical* illnesses—ones you can actually see and objectively measure. When it comes to mental health, it barely even registers as an option for a work absence.

"I feel like I'm not sick *enough* to be out of work," Luke continues. He has clearly picked up on the message all doctors receive, explicitly and implicitly.

"What does sick *enough* mean?" I ask.

"Which story do you want to hear? The one about how my attending actively miscarried, but kept working the whole time between trips to the bathroom? Or, the nurse who got into a car accident on her way to the hospital, yet worked a whole shift *before* taking herself to the ER? And then there are all the people—too many to count— who happen to be nauseated or vomiting while working, so they put an IV into their arm, grab a banana bag, and use it to rehydrate themselves, dragging the IV pole from room to room as they see patients." Luke is clearly animated now, acting out the IV dragging. He also seems angry as he lists all these examples.

"Basically, everyone around me has always come to work, no matter what, or they face consequences in the form of judgment or actual negative evaluations. Once, a med student on my surgical rotation missed work because he had pneumonia. When he came in the next day, the attending asked him where he had been admitted (meaning, to which hospital). The student said he hadn't been admitted anywhere, and the attending replied, 'If you weren't admitted, you weren't sick.' So, yeah, this system's messed up."

I wish I could say that stories like the ones Luke describes shock me. But not only don't they but also I used to buy into the idea that people who powered through bleeding or whatever illness they had were bad asses. As a med student, I remember my reaction to seeing a surgical fellow (someone who has finished residency but is doing additional training in a subspecialty, in this case colorectal surgery), pass out in the operating room. Instead of going home, when she woke up she sat in the corner away from the sterile field with a glass of water and a banana. Then she came right back into the case as if nothing had happened. At the time, I thought, *Wow!* in amazement and admiration, hoping I might be that tough someday. It wasn't until I was a chief resident and was being pushed to the brink while also hearing others' experiences that my feelings changed. But I don't say any of this to Luke.

"With all of those, to quote you, 'messed up' stories as guides, how are you supposed to know if what you're experiencing *counts*?" I ask him.

"I mostly assume it doesn't," he replies. "Wherever the stupid bar is, I can't possibly reach it. Especially with a mental health condition, and especially with a mental health condition I'm too embarrassed to talk to anyone about. I just feel so . . ."

"Guilty?" I finish his sentence because I know exactly how he feels.

"Yes, and also like people are judging me. Thinking I'm weak or somehow not *resilient* enough." He emphasizes the word *resilient* with a bit of sarcasm. "Honestly, I've been thinking a lot about the concept of resiliency lately, and I hate everything about it."

My mouth turns up in a smile because I do, too, and so do most healthcare workers. It's not that we're not resilient. Physicians have higher resilience scores than the general population, while still reporting substantial burnout. And even the most resilient physicians still have burnout.[8] Resilience isn't the problem, but it's long been incorrectly framed as the solution.

"When we start residency," Luke continues energetically, "someone comes in to lecture us on how to be resilient." I smirk a little knowing I am, in fact, the person giving all those lectures these days.

He continues, "They tell us to sleep and exercise and cook our own meals rather than eating fast food. Meanwhile, we're working eighty-hour weeks or more like a hundred, which is grueling, but we can't acknowledge that out loud because of duty hours."

By "duty hours" Luke means the 2003 national mandate that medical residents be kept to an average of an eighty-hour work week over any four-week period. This was followed by a later mandate that capped shift work for first-year residents, or interns, at sixteen hours instead of twenty-four—a mandate that was later reversed, in 2017.[9] Yes, as unhealthy as that sounds, a newly minted trainee can work twenty-four hours straight. Something only 1 percent of the American public in one survey agrees with as a limit.[10]

The limits were prompted, in part, by a fatal error in a New York hospital in 1984, when an eighteen-year-old named Libby Zion died because of what turned out to be a lethal medication interaction. The resident's misdiagnosis in her case was attributed to exhaustion and overwork.[11] When the data showed that the effects of doing work while sleep deprived are similar to those of working while drunk,[12] that only fueled the drive to change the way doctors trained and practiced.

The thing is, studies so far have shown that reforms haven't led to decreases in patient mortality,[13] meaning that the same number of patients have died however many hours residents have worked. Many in the profession argue that this means the old ways—longer hours—were fine, the implication being *I did it this way and survived and so should you*. This was even part of the reason for the 2017 rule reversal back to twenty-four-hour shifts. But I don't agree.

First, patient death should not be the only outcome that matters in these calculations. Some newer data show that senior residents working more than even forty-eight hours a week made more errors, caused preventable adverse events, and had occupational exposures. When they got up to sixty to seventy hours a week, they had two times as many medical errors and almost three times the preventable adverse events.[14] Also, creating hour limits helps prevent burnout, which should be a priority.[15] Unfortunately it's not; instead, work itself is prioritized over the humans doing that work.

Next, to add insult to injury, that work is basically cheap labor. Residents in 2020 were paid, on average, $63,400 a year, a figure that can vary by specialty, location (cost of living), and year of training; typically, it goes up very slightly each year.[16] But only about 43 percent of those residents feel fairly compensated, in part because they think their pay doesn't reflect their skill level, coupled with the sheer number of hours they work. In fact, the pay residents receive for an eighty-hour work week averages out to below $15 an hour. Even though that number is at or above minimum wage, when student-loan indebtedness (on average more than $200,000[17]) is added on, meeting a resident's cost of living becomes an even greater challenge.

———

Luke is worked up and his voice is rising. "With the hours we put in, what do they *think* is causing our fatigue? I honestly think there's this expectation that we can just keep moving, and if we don't, it's on us, not the system. Even if the train goes off the tracks and is smashing through the trees, it's like it still has to get to the next station on time. That takes precedence over everything else. Residents are just here to work long hours for low pay in a hospital that literally couldn't survive without us."

"That's a horrible feeling," I say, because I've experienced it, too— and am maybe even experiencing it now, seeing patients during COVID. It's hard to feel valued in a system that prioritizes productivity above all else. More patients, more research, more time. Even in our most vulnerable, personal moments, we can't seem to get past the medical culture that's been ingrained in us.

"And at what point do you go from being resilient to ignoring your mental and physical health needs?" Luke asks, still with passion.

"I agree with you completely. The word *resilience* is used to justify ignoring what our feelings and body tell us." *Which I do all the time*, I think. "Is there a different word you'd prefer they use?"

"I don't know—maybe *survival*."

"That's a good word. I feel like instead of stressing resiliency, we should point out that the system is horrible and broken. The problem is that systemic change takes time. So, to get through your training now, assuming you want to and it seems you do, you still have to work on coping skills or go to therapy. It's not your fault, but you do have to adapt to survive." I take a breath. "Sorry, that's me getting on my high horse about the topic."

Luke's energy matches mine as he emphatically proclaims, "Don't be sorry! You know, I really appreciate being able to have this conversation with someone who *actually* understands the system."

I smile again. This isn't the first time a healthcare-worker patient has mentioned that my specialty feels like a benefit, but it's always nice to feel helpful. Especially to someone like Luke, who was so hesitant to ask for help in the first place.

"I'm glad you feel that way. Speaking of adapting, beyond therapy, do you feel like you are at the point where you could benefit from medication as another tool to have?"

Luke hesitates. "I honestly don't even remember why medication might make a difference. I know you told me, but . . ."

"Well, it can help when you're experiencing higher levels of distress. If you feel like you're constantly at an eight, distress-wise, out of a possible ten, maybe you can get down to a three or a four. It can also help with anxiety or depression symptoms, like low mood or lack of interest in things, that may be caused by or occurring at the same time as your OCD. And it can help you cope with all the life changes you are experiencing. I think medication can be particularly good for physical symptoms, too, like any sort of heightened response you get when you're stressed and on alert, like dry mouth or a pounding heart."

"Hm, that all sounds reasonable, and definitely a lot of what you say is true for me, but I still don't know that I'm ready for meds yet— to be a person who takes meds, or rather, who *needs* meds, yet. Is that okay?"

"Yes, of course, it's your body. Just pay attention to your symptoms and come back in another month or so, and we can check in about how you are doing. And know that you can always message me if you feel like things are getting worse. I hate to say it, but it all just takes time."

He exhales deeply. "Of course, it does."

10

IT'S ABOUT 6 p.m. on Saturday evening when my pager goes off.

Four-letter word.

I'm on weekend call for the inpatient psychiatric ward, and I am responsible for any new admissions to the locked psychiatric unit in the hospital, in addition to helping the residents come up with plans for those patients. This is a responsibility I never look forward to, even though I like teaching (it's why I was chief resident—and why I work in academics in the first place). Weekend call only happens twice a year, but that's two times too many.

One of the perks of being an outpatient psychiatrist is not having to work on weekends. I typically use weekends to catch up on television shows, talk to friends (and, pre-pandemic, actually see them), and sleep. These days I'm mainly sleeping, meaning I wake up at noon if I don't set my alarm, kind of like when I was in college. The first time it happened, I was surprised, and even a little impressed. Yet as the pandemic has gone on, sleeping in on weekends has just become "what I do now." I try to not analyze it too much or to understand the why. Maybe because it lets me ignore my anxiety about my patients, or the things I have to do and for now, that's nice.

I remember a resident telling me recently how they felt guilty for sleeping in on their days off, because they should be seeing people and doing the things they can't do when they are working so hard. My advice? If you need to sleep, you need to sleep. I've been trying to follow it myself, while still knowing it's probably not the best coping strategy in the long term.

Of course, sleeping in—much less just relaxing—is virtually impossible to do when I'm on call, even if it isn't super busy. There have been weekends when I've been on and had no calls, but still can't sleep soundly, knowing that I *might* be paged awake at any point. I think that's left over from working overnight shifts in residency and never quite being able to fall asleep in the call room. The *What if I sleep through my pager?* feeling kept me aware and away from deep, good sleep then, as it does now. And if by chance I do fall deeply asleep, the anxiety dreams would torture me instead.

I notice that my heart is beating to the sound of the pager beeping, just like it did as a resident, as if it has been shocked into an unnatural rhythm. My body instantly remembers what that sound means, and it goes on high alert—more flight than fight. I look down at the number on the page, and my thoughts start spiraling. I get far ahead of myself and start to wonder about the protocol for protecting myself from COVID on an inpatient psychiatric ward, where it can be hard to get some patients to understand why they need to wash their hands, let alone keep their masks on or maintain social distance. Plus, unlike on other hospital floors, patients on psychiatry tend to be up and about, walking around, socializing over meals, and going to group therapy together. We call this the *milieu*—psychiatric-ward speak for the community interactions that help patients learn social norms and behaviors. It's an important part of the treatment, but in this circumstance it's also a big risk in terms of COVID transmission. Just stepping onto a psychiatric ward right now sounds like a potential super-spreader event. I wish I could just tap my nose and say, "Not it."

I send myself into a deeper anxiety spiral, as I find myself now perseverating about access to hand sanitizer on the units. As if I have any control over that. I think back to the time in residency when I had a middle-aged psychiatric patient drink hand sanitizer for the alcohol in it, prompting the whole unit to hide the remaining hand sanitizer to protect her. I imagine the crisis this situation would provoke now and feel my breath begin to come faster. I start searching for a bottle of hand sanitizer, opening and closing a few drawers, then dumping out my work bag. I realize I don't even have my own hand sanitizer; stores have been sold out of it everywhere.

If I'm being completely honest, just thinking about going into a hospital, hand sanitizer or not, terrifies me, and makes me empathize in a new way with Luke. I haven't seen patients in person for months now, and there's still so much we don't know about this virus and how to treat it. I can't plan for the unknown, and I like to plan. Planning brings control, and control is safe. Now, all I can do is come up with possible worst-case scenarios to be worried about. Instead of calling the resident back, I'm doomsday prepping.

One of the scenarios that most worries me, that I can't stop thinking about, is that I'll have to go onto one of the regular medicine floors, or even into one of the COVID isolation units, if the need for a psychiatric consult comes up. My asthma means that I'm a person who gets bronchitis or pneumonia when everyone else gets a cold, so thinking of what COVID could mean for my not-so-great lungs scares me. I'm really not sure that I should have to sacrifice myself for a two-weekend-a-year on-call gig just because I drew the short straw in terms of timing. Not that anyone should ever have to sacrifice themselves, I know that, but I'd rather work alone in my house, safe, behind a computer.

Just thinking of my lungs creates a heavy panicked feeling in my chest. Not quite as heavy as COVID is often described, but certainly it feels harder to breathe. My face is hot and flushed as well.

I realize I'm not just afraid of the COVID unknown but also that I'm re-experiencing the feelings so familiar to me during medical school and residency—of having to do things I don't want to do, because of "medicine" and "hierarchy," and "that's just the way it is." I couldn't say no then, and I can't now.

My predominant thought is the wish to make all my feelings stop, however possible. I'd love to sleep or run away, if I could. Instead, I turn back to my pager and find the call-back number. I take a deep breath, exhale, and dial. The resident on the other line picks up after only one ring, and I feel compelled to apologize for taking so long to call back. I don't even know how long I've been in my head.

She tells me "No worries," and then matter-of-factly goes on to explain that there is a potential consult needed on the COVID unit. A woman is on multiple psychiatric medications, and they need psychiatry to help co-manage the patient and prevent drug interactions and possible oversedation. I know I heard her say it—*COVID unit*—but I interrupt and make her repeat the words. I want to make sure I'm not somehow still creating worst-case scenarios in my head. She repeats herself, and I realize this is really happening. Four-letter word.

I wonder, *Did I somehow make this happen*? A psychiatrist would call this idea *magical thinking*, or the belief that unrelated events are somehow causally connected despite the absence of a realistic link between them. But really, medicine is a field of superstition. Just ask any ER doctor about mentioning that it's a quiet day. I believe in good and bad vibes in life and in medicine, so I can't help but ask myself if I somehow willed this nightmare scenario into existence by thinking about it beforehand. Or, if I'm being punished in some way, since I've had the good fortune to work from home until now. Whatever the reason, there's nothing I can do about it.

The resident continues to tell me about the case, and I can feel my body getting heavy and my mind getting jumbled. I hear most of what she says, but I keep missing some words here and there. I respond with a lot of "uh-huhs" because I can't seem to form words. All I manage to say is that I will protect her from exposure, of course, but add that I will also probably try to protect myself.

What I mean is that students and psychiatry residents, like the doctor who is calling me, aren't supposed to be going into COVID units. I know this, and that more experienced doctors like me are supposed to be helping them by going ourselves instead. But if I'm going to have to come into the hospital today, and go into the COVID unit, we both better be damned sure that the consult is necessary.

That's actually a valid consideration, because other types of doctors don't always understand what psychiatrists bring to the table, or maybe even what we do. It's like they completely forgot the mandatory four-to-six-week psychiatry rotation they did in med school. Among psychiatrists, there's a belief that doctors in other specialties can't handle patients' emotions and instead call us (psychiatry) to come for a consult if a person is angry or is crying. We often joke that they call and say, "What is that liquid coming out of their eyes?" It sometimes seems to me that these doctors assume psychiatrists can stop distressed patients from feeling what they're feeling simply by summoning us to the bedside. But people have a right to feelings, especially when they are in the hospital and likely scared, not to mention sick. Most of the time, their emotional reactions aren't because of a preexisting psychiatric disorder or a potentially undiagnosed one—it's because they feel unheard.

So many of my patients have told me how doctors have tried to change the subject or redirect them when they start talking about their emotional needs, or their feelings, or especially if they begin to cry. Crying is seen as a disruption to efficiency, a waste of valuable time.

Time is only part of it, though. What I think is that most doctors don't deal with their own feelings and emotions, and thus have difficulty handling other people's. I think we may even avoid conversations about emotions because they lead us to examine ourselves and our own feelings, and that's scary and makes us feel vulnerable. It's easier to avoid, or better yet, refer to psychiatry.

So, though the resident has told me that the consult is about preventing a possible medication interaction, I can easily imagine that I'm getting this call because someone is agitated or crying. I picture the medical team not wanting to deal with the tears, in part because of all the other things competing for their attention, especially on a COVID unit. I tell myself I just don't have the kindness or patience to handle that right now, especially if it means needlessly putting myself at risk. I understand how strained these teams are, and how much that compounds everyone's emotional abilities, but I don't want to get COVID because of it.

Before ending the conversation and explaining that I would call the medicine attending back instead of her playing the go-between, I say to the resident, "I don't really plan to go to the unit if I can help it because I don't think I should. I'm not exactly being a team player or the greatest example for you, but I hope I'm able to do it all over the phone, or even an iPad, if necessary."

She tells me she gets it and would do the same, validating my perception and feelings about the consult, which is not at all her role, but is helpful anyway. Sometimes teaching and support go both ways.

We hang up, and without as much as a second to catch my breath, I start crying. Sobbing is more accurate. I've never had a "diagnosable" panic attack before, but as I start to physically manifest my anxiety, I can't help but think about Naya. I feel tingly in my hands and down through my chest. I feel heavy again, this time all over, but especially in my arms—so much so that I drop my phone on the couch because I'm afraid I'll lose my grip on it. I want to curl up in a ball and tune out the world.

I lie down on the carpet, close my eyes, and say to myself, "You're okay. You *ARE okay*." And when that doesn't do anything, and maybe even makes the crying worse, I ask myself, "What would you tell a patient to do?"

I run through the potential possibilities in my mind, wishing I had made a list of what coping skills worked for me in the past, because coming up with anything helpful when I'm this incapacitated is virtually impossible. My mind is blank.

I notice my heavy breathing again, and I think, *Can I work on my breathing?* Before the thought sinks in, I know it's futile, since I'm already gasping for air. I get why my patients often laugh at that idea of using breathing exercises to calm down. Try taking a deep breath when you're so anxious that you can't breathe at all. *Next.*

For a brief second, I try to use my favorite technique of grounding myself in the moment, trying to stay in the present instead of worrying about the future. I look around the room and name five things I can see: a pillow with the state of California embroidered on it that I got as a gift for graduation from med school, the grayish carpet, my purple couch, a painting of a red classic 1950s car from my trip to Cuba, and a bottle of sparkling water. Then I name four things I can hear: cars on the street, the wind in the trees, my dog barking (she's probably scared to see me like this), and voices from the television show I was watching. Next, I think about three things I can smell: lavender hand lotion, my dog's food, and floor polish. And so on, through the remaining senses. The exercise calms me a little. The tears stop. But I still *want* to cry. *Next.*

"Can I do something more physical?" I ask. I don't have a weighted blanket, but I have stress putty and stress balls. Not only are they too far away from me right now—I'm still on the floor and they're in my home office, on my desk—but, I'd probably destroy them from squeezing too hard. I try progressive muscle relaxation instead, which is basically tightening and relaxing each of my muscles in turn. I end by scrunching up my face and relaxing it. Again, temporary relief. If someone saw me doing all this, they would probably have a lot of thoughts about my sanity. My dog seems to.

I think about taking a quick cold shower to change my core body temperature, but the last time I did that it was miserable. The water was so icy I screamed out loud. I think about journaling, but it takes too long and I'm in a rush to feel better and call the medicine attending back. Also, I don't feel like my thoughts are articulate enough to be put into words on paper.

What if I just let myself cry and be anxious? The sudden thought stops me short. Dr. Miller would love that idea—me sitting with my feelings. Naming them and letting them just be. But even the idea of this makes me uncomfortable. My feelings are too excruciating to feel.

Somehow, I convince myself to go in a different direction entirely. At our last appointment, after I mentioned that I might have to see patients in COVID units during the weekend because I was on call, Dr. Miller made a point of telling me that she was there if I needed her. She also reminded me, twice, that I had her number and could use it. It was incredibly comforting, and I told her I appreciated it, even though she wouldn't be hearing from me. I'm not the type of person who calls their therapist for help. To me, having her number felt like more of a security blanket, like the propranolol I prescribed for Naya: I assumed that knowing Dr. Miller's number was there, and I could use it, would be enough.

Now, in my panicked state, all bets were off. *I wonder if I should text her*, I think. I stop myself. It's Saturday. *I shouldn't bother her on her off time.*

I then get into a heated argument with myself about what to do. I think about how Dr. Miller wouldn't have given me her number if she didn't want me to use it; she definitely wouldn't have reminded me to use it—twice. But, I reason with myself, she also knows who she is dealing with and so realizes that she can offer, because I'm the kind of patient who wouldn't take her up on it. So, maybe it was just a gesture. Personally, I never give patients my number, but I'm also in an academic setting where they can page someone after hours if they really need help.

I go back and forth in my head, arguing the pros and cons of getting in touch or not, until I don't have the energy to keep fighting with myself. My panic attack—complete with crying—took a lot out of me, and I just need to get myself together enough to do my work. To call back the consult. To be a professional.

So, I reach for my phone and do something incredibly hard for me: I text Dr. Miller. "I think I have to go on the COVID unit and I am, um, freaking out."

Despite it being a Saturday, she responds within a few minutes: "Do you want to talk?"

Me, again questioning if I should have reached out in the first place: "Oh, I mean, I don't need to talk if it's an imposition, but I'm struggling a bit."

She texts, "Jessi, I wouldn't offer if I couldn't do it."

I stop for a moment. She is allowed to make these decisions—whom to talk to and when—for herself. She is allowed to set her own patient boundaries. It's not my job to protect her or worry about how she feels. In our relationship, as hard as it is for me to do, it's my job to prioritize me.

My text back is simple. "Yes." And she calls. As it turns out, you can ask for help and receive it.

I don't quite remember the words we exchanged, but having someone listen to me was enough. I think we often forget the value of simply being heard, of just someone's being there, not judging our feelings and instead supporting us through them. Sometimes I forget that in my role as a psychiatrist, too.

I'm relatively calm now—calm enough to call the attending back. Before I do, I take a deep breath and hope I still have it in me to avoid seeing the patient in the COVID unit (what we call "block a consult"). I was always pretty good at that in residency, respectfully asking a lot of questions to bring the attending to the conclusion they needed to reach, essentially rendering my in-person assessment unnecessary. But the skill feels like a muscle I haven't worked in a long while.

I dial, trying not to worry too much about the outcome, and I talk to the attending, whose number the resident gave me, about the patient and their question on her medications. I explain that I'm at home and could come in if they really needed me to, but that I also feel comfortable consulting about the medications over the phone. Luckily, the attending absorbs my answers and decides she doesn't need me to come in. She is thankful for the help.

After we hang up, I repeat to myself for comfort, *I do not have to go. I do not have to go. I do not have to go.* Crisis averted.

I feel lighter, like a weight has fallen off my shoulders. My breathing slows down and my heart rate does, too.

I text my therapist, just to keep her in the loop. And to say, again, "Thank you." She responds that she is happy and reminds me, again, that she's there if I need her.

Somehow that's exactly what I need to give myself permission to finally sleep.

11

MEGAN'S FACE POPS up on my screen and she mouths "Can you hear me?" as I shake my head no while smiling. After a few tries to connect the audio, I finally hear some rustling and say, "I think it's working now!" a bit too loud.

Technology issues are one of the "joys" of virtual therapy. I've had repair people come to my house multiple times to check on the internet service, and have even upgraded my package and bandwidth, but the connection still sometimes falters in the middle of a patient's sharing of something that is extremely emotionally triggering for them, such as their trauma, or serious as their suicidal thoughts. I then am tasked with asking them to awkwardly repeat something that was hard to talk about in the first place. Other times, instead of a live image of me, my Zoom screen just shows a Darth Vaderesque black box, which is particularly awkward when I'm meeting with a new patient. I've learned to accept these technical blips, but I also have my neighbor's passcode in case I need to urgently use her internet connection.

Megan settles herself and says, "Okay, good," pragmatically. I notice she is not in scrubs today; she's wearing casual clothing, including a T-shirt from a medical conference. She's also not in her car, and she looks a bit less rundown, brighter-eyed even. I'm hoping she has the day off. Maybe that's because I wish I did. She smiles, "Hi! Did you miss me?"

"Of course," I say, laughing along with her. I recall Megan's crying during our last session, just a few months ago, and admitting that she hadn't shed tears in years. I don't mention that, though I do wonder how she felt afterward. All I say is, "If I remember correctly, we were going to check in on how trying therapy was going . . ."

She cuts me off. "Can I be honest with you about something?" I nod, not knowing what to expect, but also hoping that she will always be honest with me.

Looking somewhat ashamed, she says, "I haven't gone yet."

I pause and consciously relax my face; I don't want her to perceive any judgmental looks on my part. It can be frustrating when a patient doesn't follow through on my recommendations, and sometimes that shows on my face before I can filter it. I put a lot of care and thought into my suggestions, and when a patient doesn't get on board, I feel I must not have done a good enough job helping them understand the "why" of the plan I'd put forward. Obviously, I understand the psychology of not taking action to care for yourself, and I try not to take it personally, but that can be hard, too. What makes me most frustrated, though, is when a patient stops taking their medication without telling me, and then comes in months (or even years) later, saying, "Oh, yeah, I stopped that." In those circumstances, I feel I'm not being given a chance to do my job in helping them weigh the risks and benefits. Plus, they often return because they feel badly again, or sometimes worse than before, and I can't help but wonder if we could have prevented all that by just working together in the first place.

In an effort to better understand Megan's motivations, I ask, "Because you didn't want to go to therapy?"

"No, no, not at all. I understood *why* I should go. Everything you said in our last visit made sense. It was uncomfortable to contemplate, sure, but it was perfectly logical. But my shifts in the ER got busier and other staff called out sick, so I've been picking up more shifts and working nonstop. I just have not had time to call."

She pauses and I think about how, in another situation, what she just said might seem like an excuse or avoidance. For healthcare workers, though, not having enough time is just the cold reality of the system in which they work, especially right now. Change the specialty, and even though the schedules and expectations might be different, finding time for one's mental health, especially a once-a-week appointment for therapy, is always a problem for people in healthcare. There are never enough hours in a week and never enough therapists who work outside the nine-to-five hours or on weekends. And asking for time off once a week for an appointment can really be only for a few things—and this one is stigmatizing.

"I completely get the time thing," I tell Megan. "I will say, though, that wait lists for therapists right now are *really* long, and that worries me. Another patient of mine called fourteen places and none had an appointment for three months, so as daunting as it is to even start the process, or to imagine calling fourteen places, you might just want to get on a list, if you can. You know, try to just make a few calls, and then realistically you won't be seen for a few months anyway."

"Okay. I'll put it on my to-do list for tomorrow." I wonder how long Megan's list is, knowing what my overflowing iPhone notepad looks like. "But, in the meantime," she adds, "is it okay to keep talking to you?"

"Yes, of course. That's what I'm here for."

I plaster on a smile as I answer, hoping to make her feel cared for, and because I appreciate that she trusts me and likes talking to me. Who wouldn't like that praise? But I also know that what I've just said is only partially true. I love practicing therapy and sitting with people trying to piece together their stories. Stories, after all, are what drew me to major in anthropology (I also got a master's degree in it), and then move to psychiatry. Yet I also can't see Megan regularly, or anyone else, simply to talk. I can help bridge them until they find a therapist or get off of a wait list, sure, but my schedule can't accommodate someone coming in weekly for an hour at a time. There is a shortage of psychiatrists in St. Louis, and really, everywhere else in the country. In fact, more than half the counties in the United States lack even a single psychiatrist.[1] People need access to prescribers, and so I need space and time to be one.

I try to draw Megan out and get to some meatier content. "At the risk of sounding cliché, how have you been feeling?" I ask.

She smiles slyly. "I knew that was coming. I was thinking about it before I came in. I think my answer is that I'm feeling angry."

Progress, I think to myself. One of the reasons Megan came to see me is that she was worried about her inability to feel anything. Anger is an actual emotion. I like that she is aware of it, naming it, and that she's opening herself up to me.

"Angry . . ." I echo, and pause for as long as I'm comfortable to see if she says anything else. To give her space to say something. When she doesn't, I add, probably too quickly, "Do you know where the anger is coming from?"

"I wouldn't say it comes from *one* place. It's more like . . . *many* places. The patients in the ER screaming at me that COVID isn't real as I try to save their life. The ones waiting to come in until they're really sick—too sick to have many options. I feel a bit helpless and unable to do my job well, and that makes me angry." *Me too*, I think, as I ponder the increasingly severe symptoms in my patients (or, as we call it, *acuity*), and the fact that so many aren't getting better. There's moral injury in those experiences, too.

"Being understaffed also makes me angry. So, yeah, all of it, I guess." She laughs a bit awkwardly, which maybe hints at some discomfort she is feeling in telling me this.

"I *completely* get it," I tell her. "I think people forget that anger should be paid attention to. It can be an indication of a struggle—a symptom of everything from burnout, to depression, to anxiety. We don't give it as much thought as we do sadness or worry, though, because anger isn't necessarily a clear indication that something is clinically wrong. But being pissed off can be a warning sign, too."

"I notice it, but I mostly just get mad at myself for being angry at all," Megan says. *This seems important*, I think to myself.

"Is it okay to be angry?" I ask her gently. "I know we talked last time about sadness, or at least the role of crying, but what about anger?"

"I don't think it's okay, really. I mean, certainly not to be angry *at* a patient. If I told someone a patient ticked me off, they'd understand, but they'd also judge me a little, I think."

As she says this, I get a feeling of déjà vu—not just to my reaction at the beginning of this session hearing that she hadn't taken my advice but also in remembering all the conversations I've had with Dr. Miller about this exact same dilemma. Sometimes clinical work makes me angry, like when patient messages pile up in my inbox and I'm overwhelmed. Sometimes, I spend my own therapy sessions venting about frustrating patients. We talk about it, and about my feelings, and then like clockwork I pause and, as if compelled to argue for my soul, I say, "I hope you know I don't hate my patients. I really do like them and care, I swear." Always searching for her validation. I think I also worry that my anger is incompatible with being good at my job, or at least seeming compassionate. I wonder if Megan does, too.

Megan continues, "I know friends who bottle it up at work and then end up screaming at their kids or their partners. I think people also take it out on colleagues or, more often, on trainees."

"Totally," I murmur out loud accidentally, as I start thinking about the surgeon who threw a stapler at a scrub nurse in the operating room when I was in medical school, and another who threw a clamp at a medical student. "Do you think, and this might be a slightly weird question, but do you think that somehow anger is a more acceptable emotion than some of the others you might feel during work, like sadness?"

"Yes! Not a weird question at all! Well, anger is more acceptable, at least in men." I smile in agreement. "I think anger is seen as powerful, not bad, and as messed up as it is, it's really common and so it becomes, normal, I guess?" she says.

I get where she's going, and piece together more explanation:

"Meaning some emotions are acceptable as long as they don't challenge the hierarchy, and maybe it's okay to be angry at a colleague or resident, but not someone above you?"

"YES! That exactly! I mean, I got yelled at often as a trainee myself. An attending literally told me on the first day of training that they were going to 'wipe the smile off my face.'"

"Wow."

"Yeah, I think we're taught to feel like that's just the culture of medicine, and if anyone complains or has feelings about it, they are weak or entitled." I couldn't agree more.

In a study of medical students in 2014, 64 percent reported at least one incident of mistreatment by faculty, and nearly 76 percent said they'd been mistreated by residents, including public belittlement, humiliation, and physical intimidation. Minority students were most likely to experience abuse. And again, all of these experiences were associated with higher burnout.[2]

I've been subjected to inappropriate treatment, too, perhaps most significantly during my first night on call as a third-year medical student. I was in the OR with trauma surgery, and I remember there was urgency, and chaos, and blood everywhere. I stood off to the side as the attending cracked open the chest of a patient who had just been in a serious motorcycle accident, looking for the source of their bleeding. The chaos swirled around me in a confusing way for about a half hour, when suddenly the surgeon called me from the sidelines to help: "Med student!"

As scary as it sounds, this happens all the time. It's known as the "see one, do one, teach one" method of medical-school teaching, meaning trainees are supposed to observe a procedure, then do it themselves, then teach someone else how to do it. Of course, that's usually not the case with life-or-death situations, when an inexperienced medical student can be more of an impediment than a help. Still, as surprised as I was to be called, I pushed down my nausea and tried to rise to the challenge.

The attending told me, "Make your hands like an alligator, and then put the heart in between them and pump it, like this." He showed me what to do, holding his hands to the side of the patient, explaining, "That's how you do cardiac massage; it's basically like hands-only CPR, using just your hands inside a patient's chest to massage their actual heart." I hesitated because, *what the actual fuck*, but then he took my hands and put them into the chest of the man on the table.

I did what I was told because that's what we are taught to do. I thought I had to help save the patient. As it turns out, the patient was already dead.

I found this out after the anesthesiologist looked at my attending across the table as my hands were pumping and covered in blood, and said, "It's been a while." The attending nodded, subtly. The anesthesiologist then replied, "I had a feeling when you called the medical student in." The attending smiled knowingly, and said, "Time of death, 2:05 a.m." Calling it in the moment seemed to freeze the clock in front of me.

I stood there holding the patient's heart in my hands, in shock. I kind of floated above my body and just looked down at my bloody hands. I had never seen someone die; now, this man had died while I was literally holding his heart, doing my best to save him. I had been tricked into feeling that I could, that I *had* to help him survive.

People scrubbed out, others left, and no one seemed to care about me or my feelings, which I wasn't supposed to have anyway. The other medical student in the room was jealous, and kept talking about how "cool" that must have been for me. But it wasn't cool; it was horrible, and still I knew I couldn't say anything like that out loud or I'd be judged for it. To my potential evaluators and my competition, I'd look like I couldn't cut it.

So, I buried my feelings and helped suture closed the patient's chest, then I went right to the next patient. I saw more emergencies and helped with more surgeries that night and again the next day. It's what we are taught to do. But I couldn't completely bury the hurt and anger.

I tried to tell someone higher up, in administration, and they said, "We've talked to this attending many times before. He won't change." As if "this is how he is" is an acceptable answer. No wonder change feels virtually impossible, however much younger generations try to speak up. Then, somehow, we become those higher ups who mistreat medical students, and the cycle continues.

Thinking about the hierarchy in medicine, I find myself getting angrier. I've always respected the greater knowledge of people ahead of me, but I don't think I've ever deserved to be treated poorly because of being younger and further down in rank. I don't think anyone does. Coming back into focus on Megan's anger, I ask, "And your anger lately, have you been taking it out on someone else?"

"Not unless you mean me, myself, and I."

"What do you mean by that? Taking it out on yourself?"

"Outwardly, you might not notice anything different about me. I'm still smiling and doing my job, while inside I'm tearing myself to shreds thinking about worst-case scenarios and what other people—including patients—think of me, which makes me think all these ugly things about myself. *I shouldn't be angry. Doctors don't get angry. I'm a bad doctor.* My thoughts start to spiral and soon I'm worrying that I'm going to get fired or a patient will complain, though none of that has ever happened."

I listen intently, knowing that internal critical voice well, and I follow up with, "Is that something you do a lot? Have negative self-talk?"

"Yes, absolutely, and it's happening more and more lately."

Perfectionists are not nice to themselves, but particularly in situations like working in medicine where they are in regular competition with others. Statistically, physicians are more likely to blame themselves for a mistake (self-condemnation), rather than be compassionate toward themselves (self-encouragement). These rates of self-condemnation are higher than in other fields, which helps partially explain the higher rates of burnout found in medicine. The keyword here being partially.[3]

The good news, though, is this way of thinking is something individuals might be able to change in themselves so as to feel better. To feel less helpless in a broken system, where they often feel like burnout or mental health repercussions are inevitable. By changing their mindset around mistakes, for example, it can feel like finally there is something they can work on and take control of. I'm hoping that's the case for Megan, whose negative thought spirals are a classic example of what's known as *cognitive distortions.* These mental filters and thought patterns can make it easy to fall into a negative view of reality. Most people experience these kinds of thoughts from time to time, but when they become more of a habit, they can be a sign of—or cause or worsen—anxiety and depression. I'll need to pay close attention to make sure Megan isn't depressed, and I will consider asking more about it specifically, like if she feels down, depressed, or hopeless, or is not interested in the things she used to be.

Cognitive distortions like the kind Megan describes tell us a lot about how someone perceives the world. There are about ten common distortions, and I can count four that Megan used just in our conversation today.

One is called "mind-reading." Megan does this when she assumes she knows what people are thinking when they observe her anger—and what they are thinking is unrelentingly negative. I do that, too, only for me it's reading into what it means when someone doesn't return my text or email relatively quickly: *They must be angry with me.*

Megan also uses "should statements," setting herself up with unrealistic expectations such as "Doctors can't be angry," and she "overgeneralizes," which means seeing one thing—anger—as a sign of many negative things, like being a bad doctor or person. Finally, she "catastrophizes," assuming that what is coming will be unbearable, like getting fired.

Sometimes, I'll give patients a list of types of cognitive distortions, including the common ones just mentioned, to assist them in knowing what to look for, because it's helpful when patients can stop and recognize a distorted thought themselves. Once they do, I encourage them to write down the negative thought—for example, *I'm a bad doctor* or *I'll get fired*—and notice how that thought makes them feel in the moment and what they were doing when it cropped up. This technique, known as "keeping a thought record," is a tool used in CBT (a type of therapy that focuses on the interplay of thoughts, behaviors, and feelings) to help patients identify negative thought patterns ("There I go mind-reading again") and learn to recognize the connections between those thoughts, how they feel, and their behaviors. As far as CBT skills go, this one is relatively quick and easy to demonstrate and explain, so I sometimes incorporate it into a patient's thirty-minute medication-management visit.

Granted, the exercise is harder to do than it might seem on paper, but with practice, the hope is that once a person like Megan becomes more aware of how their thoughts are distorted, they can stop judging themselves so harshly. Frankly, for someone who has never paid attention to their own feelings before, which describes a lot of doctors, just noticing these thought patterns is a huge step.

Given Megan's work schedule, I worry that keeping a thought record might feel too overwhelming and time-consuming. Instead, I give her a link to read about the different types of thoughts, and I suggest she at least read about them if she has time. Then, I recommend she try recognizing her thoughts a little more informally. I tell her to mindfully pay attention to what she's thinking, and if she notices herself being self-critical, try asking, *How would I talk to a close friend who was worried about the same thing?* I tell her to try to reframe the negative thought with that perspective in mind. We don't usually tell our friends they are horrible, or useless, or will for sure be fired—and we shouldn't tell ourselves that, either. If she can shift her thinking, even in one instance a week, she might feel a lot better. It's a concept called *self-compassion* and the evidence for it is extensive, including in healthcare professionals. As just one data point, a program in self-compassion was shown to improve well-being, reduce traumatic stress, and reduce burnout in healthcare workers for three months.[4] Honestly, the world and our jobs are hard enough, especially now. We don't need to add to that by being mean to ourselves, too.

Megan tells me she'll try to work on reframing the way she talks to herself, and being kinder.

That's all I can ask for, I think. At the same time, I hope she just doesn't get mad at herself if she doesn't do it.

12

"WELL, THE GOOD news is, I took the MCAT, finally. The bad news is . . . I got my scores." Naya's voice is tinged with sarcasm as we start our follow-up appointment. It's the kind of sarcasm that masks pain, and fortunately for her I'm fluent in it.

"Do I dare ask you to elaborate?" I say, tiptoeing into what I expect to be a really hard conversation.

"I did horribly . . . worse than in all of my practice tests," she says. Her face is impassive, her voice devoid of emotion. "The medication you gave me though, the prop one . . ."

"Propranolol, yes, lots of vowels and el's; hard to spell and pronounce for all of us. Totally annoying, " I smile.

"Yes! That was definitely helpful at lowering my physical anxiety, even if it didn't up my score." I notice she has shifted to talking about medication, probably because it's concrete and it means we can avoid talking about her emotions. I know that trick, too. I try not to take the bait.

"What do you mean by doing *horribly*?" I ask, pushing a bit, wanting to know what counts to her as *not doing well*. In my experience, many premedical students tend to catastrophize when it comes to test scores. In reality, they often get a score many people would consider good, or even better than good. But if it isn't perfect, it isn't acceptable *for them*.

"Below average for most schools. Or, as I understand it from my advisor, many schools won't even consider my application because of my scores. I'll get screened out."

My heart sinks a little with her answer. Probably because I remember when I took the MCAT, and also did worse than I had done on practice tests; advisors told me not to bother applying.

Doctors, even future ones, are not supposed to fail. That message comes directly from society and patients who, perhaps understandably, expect their doctor to never make a mistake when it comes to a patient's well-being—or life. And why should they want anything less?[1]

The trouble tends to arise when that expectation chokes off room for anyone's humanity, much less making mistakes. And when a doctor does fail, as inevitably happens, the fall can be even greater because doctors aren't prepared for the possibility of it.[2]

I wish I could comfort Naya and tell her that it will get better, except it doesn't. The tests just keep coming. Sometimes it feels as if medicine is a field of standardized tests, with another always approaching. In medical school and residency, you have to take and pass three "step" exams to be able to practice medicine. When I took them, the first one (which we all call Step 1) carried the most weight because that result was used when you applied for a residency. Then, to get your license, you have to take a board exam in your specialty, and sometimes also in your sub-specialty, and you repeat that process every ten years.

Doctors need to stay knowledgeable, but it feels like a lot, especially when someone is already struggling with the first hurdle. It's a hurdle that for Naya is compounded by structural racism, including in the tests themselves. For example, as was mentioned, many programs previously used Step 1 scores to decide who they would interview for residency spots. A study reported that, when African American and non–African American applicants were being considered for interviews, more African American applicants fell below the cutoff score needed to be considered, and subsequently they were less likely to receive an interview invitation.[3]

"So, how are you feeling about it all now," I ask, "after some time has passed to get over the initial shock, followed by staying up at night thinking about every single question you remember and what the right answer actually was?"

"I'm definitely still doing that, but much less than when I was waiting for my score and had nothing to do but perseverate over the physics equation I forgot. There's nothing I can do about it now, except retake the test. . . . Of course, I'm still anxious and I've taken the medicine almost every day to fight the panic and keep it from worsening. It helps, but I'm trying really hard to transition into an acceptance phase in my head."

"There's no use fighting the rain, if it is already raining," I reply thinking about something poignant a therapist I interviewed told me once.

"Yes . . . WOW . . . totally. I just need to find an umbrella so I can keep going. I've decided I'm still applying to medical schools, and if I don't get in, I'll figure it out. I just know I need to apply. I think waiting to apply and taking the test again would feel worse—like giving up."

"I get the desire to try. You worked so hard to get to this point already." I pause to consider the ramifications of what's about to come out of my mouth next, and I briefly consider couching it as a story about one of my patients . . . but I don't.

"Keeping in mind that I'm not trying to minimize our differences, would it help you to know that I barely passed Step 1, and my MCAT score was in the lower range of what most schools would interview?" Despite my best judgment and training not to self-disclose, I want Naya to know that sometimes things work out, even without perfect scores—though I have to fight the voice in my head warning me that Naya might now think I'm less qualified to take care of her.

She doesn't speak immediately, but I make assumptions about what she's thinking based on her facial expression, which is surprised and also pensive. *There I go mind-reading again.* At work, trying to intuit what people are thinking about me can be especially hard in a situation in which patients are thinking and feeling a lot of things. And most of the time, those things have zero to do with me.

I decide that Naya must be making the same assumption about me that I have made about her, which is that by "barely pass" I meant not getting a perfect score. That's what the dean in medical school assumed when I told her I was struggling to pass Step 1 and needed more time.

————————

It was six weeks before the exam, and I was home in Florida, ready to start studying. I had just started to have migraines, and they quickly got worse during this period, likely because of stress, though I didn't connect the two at the time. Or, maybe I just didn't want to. The migraines made it nearly impossible for me to look at my computer screen to do practice questions, but every medication I tried for the headaches left me feeling too tired or "off" to study.

There was another factor working against me, which is that I didn't study as much as I could have in medical school. I chose my school, Yale, partly for the Yale System, which features pass/fail grading, and even optional tests at times. I thought it would protect me from having to compete with my classmates and lose, which I knew I would be the case, given that I had taken the bare minimum science prerequisites as an undergrad. For many medical students, this type of pass/fail system enhances their well-being without affecting their test scores and residency slots.[4] I happened to be the exception.

Turns out, I needed tests and grades to make myself study for topics I didn't love otherwise, like physiology and biochemistry. Without tangible goals for achievement or clear markers of success, instead I tended to focus on subjects and activities I liked more, like researching the mental health of med students, or socializing, or running for (and winning) the position of class president. Ultimately, this meant I had one very big learning curve going into that six-week study period. There were some topics, like anatomy, about which I knew only the bare minimum.

With all my ducks *not* in a row, I took practice tests repeatedly, and I didn't pass any of them. About two weeks before my scheduled test date, I called our dean and said, "I can't take the test. I'm one hundred percent going to fail it. What are my options?"

She repeatedly tried to push me into taking it anyway, thinking I was concerned about not getting a high score, rather than about failing. "A lot of people call right before the test. It's just nerves. You should go ahead and take it," she said.

I understood that years of experience were informing her advice, but when I said "fail," I meant I'd actually fail the test. This is despite the fact that we were told when we applied, and then over and over again while we prepared to take time off to study, that in the history of the school, very few Yale medical students had failed. I didn't want to stand out as one of them.

I persisted with the dean. "I get that people say they failed and end up with a neurosurgery-level score, but I truly mean it: *I am not going to pass*. Plus, I'm horrible at tests; I've always been horrible at tests."

Then, to my horror, I burst into tears, which may have helped her see that I was sincere about doubting my ability, but it made me worry she might also think I was *unstable*. Somehow, though, she agreed to let me postpone the test, and so I did. I put it off for about six months and started my clinical rotations instead. To understand what a big decision this was, know that I think I was the only person in my class of over 100 students who was given this accommodation. It made me feel both grateful and embarrassed.

By the time the test came around again, my headaches had improved. I was given another month off to study, and this time I scored a little better on the practice tests, passing at least a few. And so I took the exam.

When my results arrived, I was stunned to realize that it was possible to pass with such a low score—I had made it through by what I think was the equivalent of one question. I sort of wanted to show my dean—to say, "See, I wasn't being melodramatic," but my achievement was nothing to be proud of. It's *incredibly* complicated to be a medical student who is not good at test taking, especially because some specialties, like dermatology or ophthalmology, have so few residency spots that test scores are a crucial factor in deciding who is accepted, or even who is allowed to interview. This was another moment when I was glad I wanted to be a psychiatrist.

Naya is still waiting expectantly, so I start fast-talking to prove I'm not bullshitting her about how badly I did—not that I know she is thinking this, mind you. "When I say *barely pass,* I mean I passed by, like, a single question."

What I didn't say, but what was likely also making her skeptical, is that despite my lack of test-taking prowess, I'd managed to get into two Ivy League schools, one for undergraduate college and one for medical school, which she could have discovered easily by Googling me. I've always attributed my success as an applicant to my penchant for overcompensation. Burnishing my CV (curriculum vitae) with my extracurricular accomplishments was my way of putting lipstick on a pig or, rather, saying: "Don't look at my MCAT scores—look at the fact that I got a master's and undergraduate degree in four years. Don't look at my SAT scores—look at the fact that I authored scientific publications in high school." I tried to do so much more than other students that it was (mostly) hard for people to dismiss me solely because of subpar standardized test scores. I was still wait listed for Yale Med initially, anyway.

But, there's privilege in my ultimate success. While the percentage of females enrolling in medical school more than doubled from 1978 to 2019, the percentages of medical school enrollees from Black, Latinx, and other underrepresented racial and ethnic groups remain well below the percentages of these groups in the national census.[5] I think about this often, especially with patients like Naya, and I try my best to ask the right questions, provide support and validation, and speak about it out loud and as much as I can. I may not have the same experiences as she has had, but it's important that I feel comfortable talking about inequities and racism, and that she knows I do. With only 2 percent Black psychiatrists in the United States, to truly do the best job possible for my patients, I need to acknowledge that.[6]

"Honestly," I tell her, "I'm truly horrible at tests, but I made it through somehow. Again, I know your experience is different from mine, and it includes many factors I didn't have to contend with that we've spoken about some in the past, like racism, but I really believe you can make it through, too."

I see Naya nodding and feel relieved that my self-disclosure wasn't a mistake. "That's all helpful to know," she says. "Because otherwise I'm surrounded by people doing better than me. I mean my roommate is also premed and she pretty much aced the MCAT."

"Ugh, that happened to me in high school, with a good friend and the SATs. I was taking review classes and retaking the test, and she got a nearly perfect score on her first try, no studying. It makes you feel terrible about yourself." I don't know why, but I keep self-disclosing. Maybe because Naya reminds me so much of myself at her age.

"Yes, and it definitely doesn't help my anxiety. I used to just have these peak moments of panic, but now I feel anxious all the time, and even worse during those peaks."

"What does anxiety *feel* like for you?" I ask, as it can be different for everyone. Asking to hear about someone's subjective experience ensures that I don't miss anxiety in them, even if it doesn't mimic the textbook symptoms. Being narrow in diagnostic thinking can hurt; historically, many ethnic groups, like Asian Americans, are grossly underdiagnosed as a result.[7]

"My heart starts pounding, I feel tense all over, and my mind either goes blank or it starts racing with all of the things I have to do in the future."

It's my turn to nod, as I say, "I like to think of anxiety as having one foot in the future, where all you can do is think about what's coming. It's different from depression, which is like one foot backwards, thinking and ruminating on the past. Let me ask: The anxiety you're having, does it make it hard to do things you want to be doing?"

"Absolutely. I have trouble studying, and I find myself always spiraling with the thought that I won't do well on my remaining school exams. I also haven't been hanging out with friends because I feel like if I take the time to do that, and not study, someone else will study more, do better, and get in. I can't afford the luxury of going to a movie or grabbing a drink right now."

"It probably feels like that, but we usually do better and study more efficiently if we actually take breaks." A reminder I give to college students regularly.

"I wish I could convince myself of that," she sighs. "But I don't even want to waste time with sleep! I just feel like I need to be perfect so I can win."

I completely understand where she's coming from.

Not all perfectionism is the same. In 1971, the human dynamics scholar D. E. Hamachek suggested there were two types: *normal* (or *adaptive*) perfectionism and *maladaptive* (or *neurotic*) perfectionism.[8] Normal perfectionists strive for perfection without compromising their self-esteem; their efforts can even enhance how they feel about themselves because they derive pleasure from their desire to achieve and reach their goals. They also seem to be able to sometimes ease up a bit, allowing for the occasional mistake. In contrast, maladaptive perfectionists set unrealistic goals and feel dissatisfied when they don't reach them. They regularly have thoughts about not being "good enough" or they "should" or "could" have done better. And while the adaptive type of perfectionism might help a doctor achieve good results in medicine, the maladaptive type is related to mental health issues and burnout. In one study of 169 first-year medical students,[9] for instance, those with maladaptive perfectionism were more likely to experience feelings of shame, embarrassment, and inadequacy than did their peers who did not meet the criteria for maladaptive perfectionism. They were also more apt to report moderate and severe levels of depression and anxiety. Perhaps the desire for perfection can help explain why people in the medical field tend to experience such high rates of emotional distress.

Knowing this is important to understanding the best way to support people in medicine and those who want to go into medicine. One meta-analysis found that the overall prevalence of depression in medical students was 27.2 percent,[10] compared with 8.4 percent in the United States as a whole.[11] As a practitioner who sees students like Naya on a regular basis, while I know medical school makes students much more depressed, I also know that the mental health effects of this training process start earlier, impacting whether students choose to stay in the field, or even pursue it in the first place. Premed students who experience greater burnout report a decrease in their interest in pursuing a career in medicine over time, with steeper declines in women.[12] That, and the fact that I want Naya to get better for her own sake, is why I'm glad she came to see me when she did.

"Before our visit is over, I really want to talk about your medications and whether the propranolol is enough," I tell Naya now. "It sounds like it's working really well when you take it. But with an as-needed medication, how often you need it can tell us a lot about how much you are struggling. From what you're saying, you're anxious a lot, and with the propranolol you're just chasing your symptoms. You feel badly, you take a pill, you feel badly, you take a pill, but it would be a lot better to just not feel badly in the first place."

"What do you mean? How would I do that?"

"I recommend taking a daily medication, an antidepressant, which could bring down your overall anxiety, decreasing the number and severity of the peaks." I demonstrate all this with my hands. "Ideally, it will also reduce how often you need propranolol."

"But anxiety helps me study, and I'm not depressed."

These are both extremely common reactions. "You are absolutely right," I tell Naya. "Anxiety has an evolutionary purpose, so that we can predict and run from threats.[13] For example, back when we were living among predators, it helped us say, 'That's a predator; it's dangerous to us, run!' Or, 'This is where predators like to sleep, so we probably should also run.' All the symptoms anxiety produces, even trouble sleeping, help us stay safe. And because of how hardwired and important these reactions are, medications don't bring them down to zero—more like to 3 on a scale from 1 to 10, instead of a 9 or 10, like you are now."

"Okay," she says warily. She's listening, at least.

"I would never want to give you a pill whereby you don't care about anything anymore. If that happens, let me know. It could be a side effect, and we might have to change the medication." She blinks seemingly in agreement. "And, I know you aren't depressed, but antidepressants are poorly named in that they are not just first-line treatment for depression but are also for anxiety."

"Ohhhhhh, that makes sense. I still have some more questions, if that's okay." She hesitates while I give her space and time to ask away. "If I start medication, will I have to be on it forever?"

This is one of the most common questions I get when I suggest medication to my college-student patients. (The others, perhaps unsurprisingly, have to do with interactions from drinking and smoking pot, and about sexual side effects and weight gain.) As I consider her question, I can't help but wonder if primary-care doctors are asked this when they prescribe medication for hypertension or thyroid disorders. In my patients, there's a tendency to assume that all diagnoses are temporary, and with time and a stint of medication, the patient will go back to "normal."

"Good question—and honestly one without a perfect answer. It really depends on your experience, but we usually say to take them for about six months. Keep in mind that it can take six to eight weeks to even start to notice an effect after the first dose. And the six-month prediction doesn't take into account factors such as if a person is on meds for the first time, like you, or if they have a family history of anxiety. So, a lot of it is wait and see, and then wait again, but if and when you start feeling a lot better, we can talk about it and then we can work to get off of them together."

In general, healthcare workers more so than other patients want to see the specific evidence answering their questions about psychotropic drugs. But the truth is, psychiatry doesn't always have answers. We base our decisions on the studies we do have, plus guidelines and our clinical experience. In one systematic review of patients like Naya—college students with anxiety who were on medication—those who stopped taking antidepressants had significantly increased odds of relapsing, and of relapsing faster, compared with patients who stayed on them.[14] But there also aren't good long-term data on antidepressants. In one study that looked at patients who had been taking medication for two years, their quality of life did not continue to improve, though it did initially.[15] That doesn't mean antidepressants are not good long-term medications but, rather, the data do make you question whether, if a patient's life isn't continually improving, do the medications need to be continued?

For me, the decision to stay on or go off medication is ultimately up to the patient. So many of mine choose to stop their medication once they feel better, only to find out that the medication was *why* they were feeling better. They forget, or they don't want to believe, that mental illness can be chronic, too.

To Naya, I say, "For many psychiatric meds, there aren't a million studies looking at taking them long term. Often, it ends up being a patient preference kind of thing. I wish I had more to tell you."

"It's okay. You have told me a lot. I think I'll try it," Naya says. I nod, and start going over the risks and benefits of Lexapro (escitalopram). Truthfully, there is also not a lot of efficacy data to guide me in picking one antidepressant over another, but I often choose by side-effect profiles. One drug might make you feel more awake versus sleepy or have more gastrointestinal effects. Sometimes, a bit more arbitrarily, patients just want to try a certain medication because they have heard friends have liked it (or definitely don't want one, for the same reasons). After a good risk-benefit conversation and providing them with multiple alternatives, I try to let the patient decide. Sometimes it can feel a bit like throwing darts and hoping one hits the target. Still, when it does hit, it has the chance to help significantly.

We make a plan to touch base again in a month, and as we are about to end the session, she asks me what she should be tracking to get a sense of whether her panic is getting better.

I reply as kindly and yet bluntly as I can, "Maybe just pay attention to how often you are having panic attacks, how bad they are, and how much your anxiety is interfering with your life. But try not to track all the time. I haven't found that it really helps people with anxiety to have more to obsess over. Like those fitness watches that tell you that you slept for 0.1 minute less than the night before. Not helpful. So, keep your tracking broad—don't do it every day for now, if that's okay with you."

Finally, she smiles. "I won't try to win at medication. I swear."

13

I'M SO TIRED I can feel it in my bones. My body, it seems, has given up the fight and it's a struggle to be present at all. Or even awake.

Recently, my late-afternoon appointments have been especially rough. Every day, I seem to crash earlier and earlier, now around 3 p.m. I feel myself start to yawn, though I try to stifle it by not opening my mouth. I usually get away with it, but today my patient Dennis, a somewhat verbose forty-year-old man with regular marriage strain, yawned in response to my not-quite-hidden yawn. I forgot about yawns being contagious.

Patients read into everything I do during an appointment: the words I use in response to a question, a facial expression, even taking a sip of water. A yawn definitely doesn't go over well. Patients either think you're being rude or that they're boring, neither of which helps you build an alliance with them.

Somehow, though, yawning feels like the least of my troubles. Every afternoon, I also feel my eyelids start to close, even as I blink repeatedly in hopes of keeping them open. I'm sure I look to my patients as if I have something in my eye, or I'm having trouble with a contact lens. I suppose both of those options are better than any of them thinking I'm falling asleep on them.

I have other techniques for keeping myself awake. Sometimes, I rock my chair in a slow side-to-side movement to distract myself— that is, until the chair itself begins to feel like a cradle and my sleepiness gets worse. Other times, I play with my blue, lavender-scented stress putty under my desk (I try to be subtle). Another move is to sip something, as if the act of drinking might knock some energy into me. I usually start with cold water, and if that doesn't work, I move on to caffeinated tea. You can probably measure my mental state by the number of different beverages I have on my desk by the end of the day. Today it's five.

Over the years, I've acquired multiple strategies to help me keep doing my job and doing it well. But lately they haven't been working so amazingly. Maybe that's because what I'm feeling is not the same kind of tired. It's something different.

I've even started to worry that I might actually fall asleep while a patient is mid-sentence—something I've never done before, but have heard my patients complain about from past experiences. In training, I learned that sometimes when a therapist or psychiatrist gets tired, it could be a protective response to whatever the patient is discussing—a form of dissociation. As if the mind is taking a vacation from the body, when it all becomes too much. With everything patients have been telling me lately about their work on the frontlines, this makes sense. I would rather sleep and avoid than feel any of it, or maybe they would, and that feeling is transferring to me.

As much as I try to keep actively listening, nodding, and making affirming noises, my mind continues to protect me, and it wanders or even goes completely blank. Sometimes I realize that I've missed entire sentences and have to ask the patient to repeat, which I don't like doing, either.

With Dennis, I knew I just needed to make it through to the end of our appointment. Ten more minutes. So, I turn to my last resort, a trick I learned in medical school: Using the fingernails of one hand, I pinch the nailbeds of the other hand as hard as I can. It's something doctors do to patients to assess brain function and whether a patient is in a coma. It is quick and painful, and it definitely wakes me up (because I'm not, in fact, in a coma). As I pinch, I want to yell, but push it down.

Still, the effects lasted only five minutes, and then I have to do it again, harder this time, under the table, being careful not to wince. It does the job, but after a brief feeling of relief, I mostly feel guilty and concerned that he has noticed my fatigue and thinks I'm a bad doctor. *Good doctors don't yawn or seem sleepy.* Fatigue is okay, even a sign of hard work, but a patient should never see it. That's a weakness.

Usually, after I see my last patient of the day, I spend another ninety minutes or so writing my patient notes, which are mandatory. This afternoon, as is happening more and more frequently, I simply can't look at my computer for another minute. Instead, I turn on a mindless sitcom, hoping to just relax. *I'll do the notes later*, I think. The next thing I know, it's dark and I realize that I have been sleeping for three hours, straight through dinner. Napping on the couch would be fine, in theory, if it meant I could still fall asleep at night. But these unintentional late-afternoon naps have been keeping me up well past midnight, sometimes to 3 a.m., which means I'll be tired again tomorrow, when the alarm goes off at 6:15. It's a vicious cycle: nap, then stay up late, then feel horrible again the next day, then nap again, and so on. It violates every rule of good sleep hygiene. "Well, of course you're tired," I can hear Dr. Miller saying. It's a sign of therapy working when you internalize the doctor's voice. I guess that's a bright spot.

Yet, as much as I know these long afternoon naps aren't particularly good for my well-being—something I tell patients all the time and have been discussing with Dr. Miller since I started sleeping in like a college student, months ago at this point—I actually can't fight them. I wonder, as Dr. Miller has pushed me to think about in our more recent sessions, *Is my sleep avoidant or restorative?* The truth is, at this point, it's both. I need sleep, and I haven't slept, so it's restoring a deficit, at least partially. But I'm also sleeping to obliterate the reality of my job and the constant negative cycle of the news, even if I'm not making the choice consciously. Avoidance can temporarily be nice, but now I know it also means I am probably not getting what I need to feel better, like community.

Whatever the cause, I feel I'm losing control, and not just of my sleep habits. I'm quicker to snap at people, or to cry. The tears fall easily during daytime talk shows, commercials, and even silly rom-coms on Netflix. Anything *remotely* heartwarming, and the tears start coming. I don't like being so emotional, so to save face I've started avoiding friends and family—and by that, I mean avoiding their calls, emails, and texts. I'm usually the one who always has their phone on hand and texts back immediately. Now, I ignore my messages. For days.

I'm just not sure I can handle whatever it is people might want from me. My friends and I tend to have real conversations—the kind in which we tell each other what we are going through and support each other through it. I was a supportive person long before I was trained to be; my training just made me better at it. Understandably, my loved ones assume I'll be there now, in the midst of a global crisis, the same way I was before. But I can't do it. Just a few days ago, a friend texted me to ask if I could give a talk to her women's health-care group, and my first impulse was to throw my phone across the room. I stopped myself, somehow, and have barely picked up the phone since. I'm worried that if I respond to anyone, I'll have more to carry . . . and there's just no space left inside of me.

Eventually, though, guilt pushes me to look at what I've been missing. I take a deep breath and start scrolling through my backlog of messages, about fifty deep, skimming first to decide who, if anyone, I will respond to. I feel proud of myself for at least *trying* to set a boundary.

One of my friends has texted multiple times, concerned by the unusual delay in my response. I immediately wonder if I've set the bar too high in terms of how available I make myself. She is also a psychiatrist and is reading my behavioral pattern as a sign of my mood. She is correct, as usual, but I don't want to go into that with her right now. I text back, "I'm alive. Just tired." She immediately responds with a thumbs up. I hope that satisfies her for now.

I scroll down and also see a text from my mom. Instead of texting back, as I usually do, I call her. We haven't talked on the phone in about two weeks, because I simply haven't had the energy to speak. I talk so much during my work that talking after hours feels like an impossibility.

We catch up briefly, then, as moms do, she asks, "Are you okay?"

Everyone keeps asking, so of course my mom would, too. "Yes, I'm just really tired," I say again, pointing the finger at fatigue as the only reason for my lack of communication. I think that's easier to say than an actual feeling like angry or sad, as that invites a bit more commentary and concern.

"I can hear it in your voice." I wonder if I sound hoarse, or sick, or sad. Whatever it is, I must not sound okay. "Also, it's been a while," she points out. "We talked more when you lived across the country." She is referring to the fact that even when there was a three-hour time difference between us, and I was a resident with terrible hours, I still managed to stay in better touch.

I instantly feel guilty. Moms are good at that, especially Jewish ones. Still, in college and medical school, I called home multiple times a week; now, until lately, I clock in at about once a week, so I can see how this change might be a red flag.

"I'm so sorry, honestly; it isn't about you at all. This pandemic is a lot and people are a lot. I'm just exhausted by the end of the day, listening to and absorbing everyone's stuff. I'm clearly not dealing with it as best as I can." "Avoidance," I hear Dr. Miller say in my head. Out loud, I tell my mom that I'll do better.

I think she understands, but as she reminds me, *mothers worry*.

It's beginning to seem like everyone is worrying about me, so maybe I should be, too. This emotional and physical exhaustion isn't sustainable.

"Well, what do you think your body is trying to tell you?" Dr. Miller asks a few days later, during our scheduled Thursday session.

"That it needs to sleep," I say, with a slightly sarcastic smile.

She pauses, then slowly says, "That's true, sleep is *clearly* important to your mental health, but what else could it be?"

"That I'm working too hard? I think that's part of it. I'm doing a lot right now, and I'm wearing too many hats, like taking on more patients and extra writing, and saying yes to giving interviews to the media, and of course doing lectures. I feel like I can't say no to any of it."

Dr. Miller nods, taking it in, "You have a lot of reasons to be tired, but you've been tired before, you've even been overcommitted before, so what's different now?"

"It's hard to explain, but it just feels different. I feel different. I'm scared something is really wrong with me, because I can't fight my fatigue. It's not an 'I worked long hours, or my job is emotionally exhausting' kind of tired. It's like my body is just done. . . . I'm also worried my patients can see it, and that it's starting to affect my work. I mean, I still show up and do my job every day, but even my boss told me I need to take some time off. So, that felt like something bad."

Dr. Miller asks, "Your boss said those exact words?" I pause and notice that I feel a bit on edge. Dr. Miller knows I have a tendency to perceive judgment in conversations where there really isn't any. My friends tell me that, too. So, she's right to ask for specifics, but it still feels as if she is somehow questioning the veracity. I tell myself to calm down, that she's pushing because she cares and wants to help me notice my thought patterns. I feel slightly calmer.

"I don't remember, honestly; let me read you the text chain." I go to the wall where my phone is plugged in and I grab it so I can find the messages and start talking while scrolling. "It was one of way too many messages I hadn't responded to, so it's taking a second.

Sorry . . . okay, found it! So, this is a friend, who also happens to be my clinical boss, meaning she runs the outpatient clinic. There are a few texts before this one, catching up, and then she asks me, 'Do you have any time off planned? I think you should take some.'

"I responded, 'LOL. Do I seem like I need to?' And she says, 'No, but things are only going to get worse. People need us a lot right now and we're busy, and before you know it, fall will be here and it's back to school and there's heightened distress, and then winter, and depression season, so it's best to plan your time off now.'

"I reply, 'I'm taking a day for a virtual talk I'm giving.' To which she said, 'Time off to do talks does not sound like time off to me.'"

Dr. Miller's somewhat neutral expression turns into a smile as she says, "I believe we've had that conversation before." I smile back. "So," she pushes on, "how did you feel about that conversation?"

"I think my first reaction was that it must mean I'm screwing up in some way, or that it's obvious I'm struggling. I noticed I was getting really defensive, and then I started to think about the evidence: I'm still doing what I need to do—seeing all my patients and writing up my notes, which she can see on her end. Sure, I'm a bit shorter with my email responses, but I doubt she'd notice that. So, it must be that she's just concerned because I haven't responded to her as quickly as I usually do. Like everyone else has been."

"Or maybe she is saying the same thing to everyone, and it hit differently because you're struggling right now?"

"That, too. I think even on my best days, any somewhat negative feedback even in a sea of positive feedback can do that to me. Let alone me, now."

"Okay, so fear of judgment aside, what do you think about the time-off suggestion?"

"Who doesn't like time off? But I don't see how I could possibly do that right now. People are not okay, our clinic is busy, and I don't have an excuse to be off. I'm not sick."

"Do you have to be sick to take time off?"

We've had this conversation before, too, but I feel justified in my response: "Right now, with everything going on in the world, I feel like I do need a really legitimate reason to take time off. The COVID bar is high. If I can work, I will, even if maybe I shouldn't."

I look at her to gauge her facial expression. It doesn't say much, other than that she is taking it all in, so I continue. "Plus, I'm sure you've realized this by now, but this 'working no matter what' value is a longstanding, training-engrained thing. Basically, I'm a machine who works, not a person who works. I'm not sure you can *fix* that part of me. . . . Not to mention that I'm not sure I even deserve to take time off. I'm not a frontline worker or anything."

As I say this last part, I realize just how guilty I still feel about being able to stay at home, protected, even if it's what I also want. Somehow, I have to punish myself for my advantage. Going to work no matter what and taking on extra work seem to be my methods of choice.

Dr. Miller looks at me with care. She doesn't say anything, so I prod, "I mean, do *you* think I need time off?" Honestly, part of me is hoping she'll just tell me to do it so I have no choice: *therapist's orders*. Though I worry I'm too far gone for any vacation—however long—to help much. I can't help but ruminate on the look on the face of my patient James on Monday, when he told me that I'd met him before. His hurt, and better yet my feelings in the moment and since, the anger, guilt, and anxiety, keep bubbling up. I don't know why I haven't told Dr. Miller about it yet. Maybe I'm embarrassed she'll think I'm a bad doctor, too.

Without thinking, I blurt out, "What if all of this has nothing to do with taking time off? What if *I'm* the problem?"

"Wow, well that's a doorknob moment." Dr. Miller says bluntly, as her eyes lift up from looking, presumably, at the clock. This concept is the habit some patients have of waiting until the last moment of the appointment, when we are nearly exiting the door, to reveal something crucial. Some argue that patients wait because, unconsciously, they don't want the therapist to have time to talk about the extremely painful topic, but they know they should tell them anyway. It's like I know that forgetting a patient is important and clearly bothering me, but I also don't want to deal with the feelings it brings up. Sometimes I know when I'm "doorknob momenting" myself and I try to decide if I want to have the conversation about why it took forty-nine minutes of a one-on-one visit to finally say the important, painful, thing out loud. But, this wasn't one of those times.

Dr. Miller gently asks me for more details.

I quickly rehash what happened with James. The emotionally laden tale of how, for the first time ever, I forgot a patient I'd met a month earlier, and I reintroduced myself. I tell Dr. Miller I've been replaying the moment ever since when James said, "I *know* you, Dr. Gold."

I add, "I never want to hurt anyone. I knew I wasn't at 100 percent, but I figured my 50 percent was better than nothing, and maybe better than a lot of people's 100 percent. I'm not so sure that's true anymore." For the first time, I'm worried my own shit could be interfering with my work with patients.

I look over at Dr. Miller whose face stays neutral, following along until I finish. She then takes a deep breath and says, emphatically, "I just want you to know that this is representative of all that is going on with you, rather than an indicator of you as a psychiatrist, or person. I know you care about your patients tremendously."

I start to cry, and truly allow myself to. I needed to hear that. "Thank you," I mouth.

She's basically hugging me with words through the screen as I wipe my tears on my sleeve. I knew she'd help me figure it out, or rather, figure *me* out.

"Now," she says, "I don't want to tell you what to do, but it seems like you could *really* benefit from some time away from work and the notifications and screens. When is the last time you took off for vacation, not work?"

"More than eight months ago? I went away at Christmas with

some of my family. It was nice. But even if I did take time off again, where would I go? Everything is closed." I say this as a last-ditch effort to stay put. I appreciate Dr. Miller's concern, but I get it why so many of my patients aren't using their vacation days now. Why bother?

"Do you have to go somewhere to take time off?" Dr. Miller asks. "Couldn't you stay home?"

"I mean I *couuuuuld*, but then I'd be having people cover my patients for what? For sitting in my house, watching TV?"

"Yes. Or, for doing anything you wanted to do." I knew she had a point, but it was hard for me to absorb it.

"Your vacation days are yours to do whatever you want with. Do other people always tell you where they are going or why they are taking off?"

I think long and hard about all the times I have covered for colleagues, and it hits me that of course I mostly had no idea what they were doing on vacation or what their symptoms were if they were sick. Why did I feel the need to explain myself? What if I just didn't?

"You're right," I tell Dr. Miller. "But if I don't go away on vacation, and I just stay home, is there something positive I should be doing with my time?" Clearly, I'm still trying to get an A in therapy.

She suggested I consider putting away my phone and computer, maybe even leaving them with my neighbor for some good peace and quiet for at least a day. I bristle at the thought, knowing I haven't even been able to walk my dog without playing a podcast, her last no-device suggestion for me. Still, I know I need to do something different, and I trust her. I know she wouldn't give me more work that isn't worth it, knowing full well I have enough on my plate as is.

She can tell I look uncomfortable and adds, "I know you don't love being alone with your thoughts. This is different, though. I didn't say you couldn't do anything, just that you couldn't be on your phone, or looking at any screen, including a television or a computer."

"Might not be the most relaxing vacation . . ."

"It might be a necessary one, though. You know how on the Sabbath, observant Jews take a day of rest and don't use electronics?" I nod. "I think they have a good thing going."

A day or so of real rest, I think. Sometimes I hate it when she's right.

14

"I'M GETTING READY to go back to work," Janet tells me on the computer screen. She's in a baseball hat and a T-shirt, but what stands out most for me are the dark circles under her eyes. She has makeup on, but they're still visible, reminding me that even if she says she is "okay," it has clearly been a few hard months for her. "Can you believe it? My maternity leave is almost over."

"That was fast!" I interject, still having no concept of the passage of time, but also knowing that maternity leave in the United States, and especially in healthcare, is far too short—generally eight weeks for attendings, six weeks for residents, and anywhere from six to twelve weeks for nurses like Janet. If I'm counting correctly, that means her baby must be seven or eight weeks old by now. No wonder she hasn't been in touch.

"Yes! I feel like I just got settled at home, and now I have to go back again." I see her shaking something off camera, and I hear the faintest mewing sound. I ask, "Is that . . . ?"

"Yes, this is Gabriel . . . Gabe." She shifts the camera so he is in plain view.

I get really excited. "Hi, Gabe! It's nice to meet you!" Even though I don't have children, I do like other people's children. There's something I find especially comforting about seeing a baby start to smile amid everything going on in the world. Maybe it's that babies are oblivious to it all. Maybe I'm even a little bit jealous of that oblivion.

Janet keeps rocking him ever so slightly in his bassinet, but does not pick him up. "Alright," she says. "I think he'll be okay now."

I like this little window into her life that telehealth has provided me, though I know that because of Gabe, as well as her daughter, who I think is seven years old now, there will likely be more interruptions. It happens with every patient, sometimes from my end. I may not have kids, but my house is full of unexpected noises and visitors, from package-delivery guys, to my dog barking, to lawn mowers buzzing outside the window.

I smile, and ask, "So, obviously a lot has happened. Catch me up; how's it all been?"

"Stuff's been . . . hard since Gabe's birth. Okay, maybe even before. I can't remember when I saw you last, but I know I was still pregnant. I ended up working almost until the very end, until I couldn't anymore. I did that last time, too, with Maddy. Actually, with her, it's kind of a funny story, but I went into labor during a shift. Like, I started having contractions while I was doing chest compressions on a patient. As I went up and down, and up and down, the whole time I was afraid my water would break, but I didn't say anything. I didn't even think about saying anything. It simply didn't occur to me to be, like, 'Oh, I'm in labor, I should go now.' That's not what a nurse does. I finished helping the patient, who survived, then walked upstairs to get myself admitted to the hospital. I was calm and collected, and somehow I felt able to manage everything, even though I'd never given birth before. But not this time. All my previous experience and serenity went out the window. Truly, nothing can prepare you to do this in a pandemic."

"It's not just a different pregnancy; it's a very different birth experience now, isn't it?"

"Oh, yes, like no family was allowed in the hospital except my husband, and I was terrified of my newborn contracting COVID. I remember just being in the hospital, overwhelmed and anxious about it all. My husband was scared, too, and upset to see me so upset."

"I can imagine."

"To add to it all, Gabe was born when the George Floyd protests were happening all over the country. I remember one morning we were doing skin-to-skin contact, and I looked up at the television and was, like, 'Oh, my God, what world am I bringing him into?' I couldn't stop watching the video of George Floyd's murder, then the protests, and the fires, and the police violence. I've never been religious in my life, but suddenly I was scared and thinking, *This is Book of Revelation shit*. I started to pray because there was nothing left to do for him—and all of us. My overwhelm was through the roof. I sometimes still feel that way."

I nod slowly. "Religion can definitely be a source of coping and comfort. I'm glad it's helped you, even if it came out of fear." Studies agree: Positive religious coping, or a strong relationship with or faith in God, was associated with lower anxiety and more positive outcomes in the setting of COVID,[1] including in international studies of nurses.[2] Even though sometimes people pit medicine against religion, many hospital chaplains have told me that healthcare workers are turning more often to them for help, and not just for their patients. In one 2021 study, 56 percent of chaplains described an increased need for and facilitation of emotional and spiritual support for healthcare staff.[3] In a way, this further illustrates the rising demand for, but continued stigma associated with, mental health care in healthcare workers: Asking a chaplain feels safer and less formal, and ultimately less stigmatizing, than a visit with someone like me.

I continue trying to better understand Janet's current level of distress. "And, what have you been experiencing lately, besides general worries about the world?"

"It's still hard, but maybe a different hard. While I was pregnant, I was afraid I'd get sick and die of COVID, but now I'm afraid I'll get COVID and kill my kid." She looks down and her eyes well up. "This isn't easy for me to say, and I haven't really talked about it with anyone, but I won't even let myself hold Gabe. I don't want to risk infecting him. So, I just sit there, face-to-face with my baby, and feel like a mess. There's no joy. My husband tells me 'You won't hurt him, it's fine,' but he could say that 1,000 times and I can't let myself fully believe him. Outside of daily, or hourly, COVID testing, I don't know what can be done."

"That sounds like it would be a huge challenge, and maybe even one that makes you feel like you aren't doing what you're supposed to as a mother?"

"Oh, yes, Dr. Gold, that's so spot on. I can't tell you how many nights I've laid down next to Gabe with a mask on, and I get this feeling that I shouldn't be around him at all, that I don't deserve to be his mother, and I just start to cry. That's part of why I'm back here."

Her symptoms are starting to sound like postpartum depression, which I know she had after giving birth to Maddy; it's part of why she stayed on her medication during her second pregnancy and connected with me in the first place. In one study, women who experienced postpartum depression with their first birth were up to forty-six times more likely to experience it with later births.[4] Even without the added stressor of COVID, it makes sense that her mood would once again worsen during this post-birth period.

I think about her risks and how glad I am that she established care with me early on, as it would likely feel impossible for her to do it now, with her new baby and returning to work, and of course her depression. A person's not being able to get appointments easily is one of the things I hate most in my field. When you're depressed, it's hard to get motivated to try to get an appointment in the first place, and if you are anxious, it's tough to bring yourself to talk on the phone to anyone, let alone a new doctor. Adding to all this, it's harder than ever to get an appointment now, when so many people need help. But we keep asking, well, expecting people to find their own care, like it's nothing at all.

I add, "And I imagine that having to go back to work is making it all worse."

"Incredibly. Not just in the obvious way that I'll be more exposed to COVID, which exposes Gabe more, but also it felt like such a luxury to be able to get away from everything during my maternity leave, including COVID. I don't have that luxury anymore."

"How did you manage to block out everything?" I ask, wondering if she had some secret way to compartmentalize that I haven't learned yet.

"Every time the pandemic came up on the news or on Facebook, my anxiety would skyrocket, which made my negative thoughts and depression even worse. It was a clear trigger, so I decided to stop reading things and watching things, and kind of stay safe with Gabe, and Maddy, and my husband in the bubble that is my house. I barely left because we didn't *need* to leave. I got bored and lonely sometimes, but at least I didn't have to think about COVID. And at work . . ."

"It's all there is."

"Yep."

"With going back to work, what do you worry most about?"

"Being exposed to all of that trauma again."

One of the things I've learned as a psychiatrist is that trauma—and whether or not something is traumatizing—can be in the eye of the beholder. People tend to use the word a lot, and there are a number of mental health professionals who argue that it's overused—maybe because of TikTok and other social media. I believe that feelings about an experience are always valid: If someone feels hurt, they *are* hurt. Too often, our discussions of trauma are limited to things like war or assault, but trauma is so much more than that.

Mental health professionals tend to talk about "Big T" and "Little

T" traumas. The first are the ones I just mentioned: catastrophic, life-threatening events, like experiencing a natural disaster, war, sexual violence, or serious injury. "Little T" traumas are smaller-scale events that are not typically life threatening, but are stressful nonetheless. They include things like moving, divorce, job loss, or financial emergency that can cause significant disruption in emotional functioning. By definition, however, they don't typically cause post-traumatic stress disorder, otherwise known as PTSD.

To be clear, it's normal to have symptoms like sadness, anxiety, or stress after something traumatic occurs. And though about 70 percent of people will go through at least one traumatic experience in their lifetime,[5] most of them won't develop PTSD (only about 6 out of every 100 people do).[6] Those who do develop PTSD must meet strict diagnostic criteria[7] to receive that diagnosis, from four different symptom categories. These categories include: intrusive symptoms, like experiencing flashbacks to the trauma; avoidance symptoms, like avoiding people, places, and activities that might trigger a memory; changes in cognition and in mood, like forgetting aspects of the event, or having negative thoughts or feelings about oneself, including guilt or shame; and shifts in arousal and reactivity, like irritability and angry outbursts, being startled easily, or behaving in a self-destructive way. In one study conducted pre-pandemic,[8] the reported prevalence of PTSD in nurses (28.4 percent) far exceeded the prevalence in the general U.S. population (7 to 8 percent), and even wartime veterans (10 to 20 percent). Like so many things, COVID didn't create the problem (PTSD in nurses), but it did compound it.

Healthcare workers can also experience trauma as a result of indirect exposure to a threatening event, like hearing patients' stories (as is common in mental health professionals) or delivering bad news. They can then develop something called secondary traumatic stress (or vicarious trauma), and it looks a lot like PTSD. In many ways, it is the cost of caring, which runs counter to burnout, which is the cost of an unsupportive workplace.

Based on Janet's subjective use of the "T word," I know I need to do a deeper screening for PTSD than I did on her intake. I want to see if she might have it on top of her depression—something that is actually pretty common: Almost half of people with PTSD also suffer from depression.[9]

"When you say *trauma*, what do you mean?" I ask, plugging into the subjectivity of the word.

"Before I left for maternity leave, everything about work was distressing and disturbing. Even after being away, I was thinking about it more than I'd like, and now that I'm about to go back, the thoughts are getting even more frequent. I was filling out some HR paperwork and suddenly I found myself remembering a case I had back in March, with a husband and his wife. He came in with COVID, and then she did a few days later, both of them really sick. Her room was across the hall from his, and they had maybe five kids and their youngest was Maddy's age.

"One day he was getting better, and I said, 'Listen, if you continue to get better, we will take you across the hall to your wife, and you can hold her hand.' He reached out, touched my arm, and said, 'Do you think that's possible? That I can see her?' And I said, 'Yes, we can roll you across the hall, if you get a little better.' That day I left work and it felt like a win, like I was really helping him, and I felt a real sense of purpose.

"But that night, while I was home sleeping, he died. Instead of him getting to see his wife, they wheeled her across the hall after he died, and let her sit there with him. When I think about it, I'm back in that moment; the sights and even the smells are so real, and that feeling of loss."

I make a note that this sounds like a flashback to me, one of the classic intrusive symptoms of PTSD. Just having this symptom, or any of the others, doesn't necessarily mean a person has PTSD; to count, the symptoms need to last for more than a month and cause significant distress or problems in a person's daily functioning.

"That's a lot to hold," I say, pointing out that an experience like this would be hard for anyone.

"I still cry when I think about it." She wipes away tears from her eyes. "And it's just one of the many horrible stories." Janet's gaze turns unfocused and she looks heartbroken, as if she is remembering them now.

As she pauses, I secretly hope she won't tell me more, both because she doesn't need to further expose herself to the trauma by repeating the details and, frankly, because I don't need to be exposed, either. Often, when I hear detailed stories of patients being really sick or dying, it's hard to stay detached. As with Janet, I sometimes feel the urge to stop the person from telling me before my emotions overwhelm me. I can also feel myself disconnecting or tuning out slightly— for self-protection.

I've even noticed that I feel agitated going into an appointment with a patient I suspect will be emotionally difficult. I've wondered if this is a self-protective reaction, too, just as fatigue can be, because it might be easier to feel agitation than sadness. It isn't about the person doing the talking. It's about helping myself, while still doing my job and not being "found out" as the psychiatrist who let her own emotions cloud her reactions. It's about trying not to have secondary trauma, even if sometimes my whole job can feel like secondary trauma. I still have to try.

"Thank you for trusting me with your experience, even if it's hard to talk about," I muster. I'm hoping to validate her sharing, as people disclosing trauma can often feel additionally traumatized by the reaction of the person they disclose to. "Do you notice you usually try to avoid thinking or talking about work or things that remind you of it?" I ask, screening for avoidance symptoms of PTSD.

"I mean, I'm in luck because I'm not at work right now."

"But what about the anticipation of it?"

"I definitely think about not going back, or what excuses I can come up with to not go in every day. I'm an introvert, and it reminds me of how I sometimes used to make plans, then hope the person would cancel so I didn't actually have to go through with them. That's how I feel with work."

"I know what you mean." I'm not an introvert, but I've also wanted to come up with excuses to cancel plans and not go to work, especially lately.

Janet sighs. "I think I also worry that work won't bring me joy anymore."

I ask her to explain.

"Honestly, before I went out for maternity leave, I'd already reached this point where something in my attitude had changed. Part of my joy in the job has always been about seeing patients and taking care of people, and kind of jokingly, wanting to fall a little bit in love with one patient every shift. That's always been my little goal: to find something, some little nugget about somebody who is essentially a stranger. Like, I met a lady years ago, and I still think about her; she told me that she designed race cars. This little old lady. How cool is that?

"But, right before I went out to have Gabe, I realized that I didn't want to *know* anybody anymore. It's almost as if a switch had flipped, and instead of wondering, *How can I love this person?* I was thinking, *Is there any way I can care for these people without getting to know them?* And that's not me. That's not me at all. And I worry I'll still be like that."

"Well, what do you think the change was about?" I probe, thinking if she understood the root of it, maybe she could address it more head on.

"Well, I realized that I wanted to stop asking about them because I didn't want to mourn them when they passed. It was getting to be too much."

Janet, just as I do, and as so many of my patients do, is trying to protect herself by distancing and by tamping down her empathy to prevent experiencing grief. Grief is a hard emotion for healthcare workers to process. As they are not a friend or family member of the deceased patient, they often wonder if they even have the right to mourn. Not to mention that there are no rituals to support this kind of grief. Most healthcare workers I talk to aren't sure they would be welcome at a funeral, for example, and only a few have chosen to attend. It feels very isolating.

The sheer magnitude of death and hospitalization only makes this harder. By May 2020, the *New York Times* front page featured the names of the first 100,000 people to die of COVID,[10] a number that would double by the end of the first six months. Janet wasn't exaggerating or catastrophizing; she really had witnessed all of it. It's an experience many of us heard about from the mouths of healthcare workers, but can't really tangibly imagine, even if we try.

I continue, "From my perspective, I don't think you quite meet the criteria for having PTSD yet, which you might have noticed I was asking about. But the keyword is *yet*. I think we need to pay a lot of attention to your symptoms, to what your body tells you, with you going back to work. To all of it."

"I can do that."

"I also recommend increasing the dose of your medication in anticipation of returning to work again, just to give you a little added buffer."

She nods. "I'd really like to stay where I am for breastfeeding, but I hear what you are saying. I've had a lot of conversations about taking medication while pregnant and breastfeeding, and I understand that the risk is pretty minimal. So, if you think it's best, I'll do it."

"I do."

She nods, again, "Okay, I trust you." Words that mean a lot more to me than she probably even realizes.

I add, "And . . . I'm not trying to be overly positive or naive, but I really hope the time away from the hospital will help you get your spark back. I know you weren't on vacation, but you did get a break from COVID. I hope you find the thing that makes you, *you*—with patients and as a nurse. You seem like you are so good at your job, and care so much. Patients could really use someone to ask about their hobbies and want to know who they are as people, especially now."

I didn't mention this part to Janet, but something is missing with me, too—my *je ne sais quoi*. I haven't even had the energy to make jokes anymore.

I really hope that I will get it back. But though I try to be optimistic for Janet, it's harder to be optimistic for myself. I worry that this is just me, now.

15

"I'M STILL FEELING off, and I'm pissed about it," I tell Dr. Miller. I've just returned from taking some time off, as she and my boss suggested, and she wondered how it felt. I realize I'm angry, mostly because it wasn't the silver bullet I desperately needed. "It's just, I did what you said, and even booked a bed and breakfast for a few days with my dog."

"Yes, I remember getting your out-of-office message. I was glad to see it."

I feel a bit lighter instantly and recall the message Dr. Miller had sent back. She told me she was happy that I was taking care of myself, which felt like finally getting a gold star in therapy—a dose of validation I very badly needed to quiet the guilt of time off.

"Well," I continue, still bolstered that she has remembered my message, "I listened to your advice and didn't work the whole time I was away. I just hung out and even tried to read for fun—no mental health, feminism, or advocacy-themed books, as discussed, either. I really should feel more relaxed now but clearly . . . " I gesture to my face and the tears that are starting to form in my eyes.

She sighs quietly. "Truthfully, did you think a long weekend would be enough for a complete reset?"

As she says this, I think of all the times my patients have sought out quick fixes, as if feeling better happens on demand. Sometimes, that desire to feel better instantly leads some patients to try anything possible to cope, from a sham treatment to binge eating or drinking.

A drink after work is just a drink, until it's a drink (or two or three) after work every day for months.

I smile a little smile. "Well, I *hoped* it would. Honestly, hope is hard now, so I take it where I can get it."

"I can understand that, but try thinking about it like this," she says, shifting forward. I feel myself sitting up too, mirroring her, suddenly extra-attentive. "It's like you are a leaky boat full of water. Taking a few days off is like bailing out a few pailfuls. The boat might float a little lighter, bobbing higher on the surface, but in the end you're still a leaky boat in the middle of the ocean."

I pause to take this in. Dr. Miller is so good at metaphors, and they always stick with me. "So, what you are saying is . . . I'll eventually go back to sinking."

"Precisely. A few days off is just a temporary fix. It's not that you shouldn't have taken the time, but it doesn't negate how much water was in the boat to begin with. It doesn't fix the problem."

Just like yoga, or a massage, or other self-care solutions aren't going to fix a person's toxic workplace or bad relationship, I think to myself cynically. That isn't to say these things can't help at all (who doesn't love a massage?). There's also evidence that techniques like mindfulness do work really well for some people.[1] The problem is, they are constantly suggested as cure-alls, as if they are enough to get someone through a major life crisis. To me, when someone suggests finding time for self-care or gives me advice on coping, it feels a bit like they're saying, "So, you worked eighty hours listening to everyone talk about the pandemic this week? No worries, a deep breath will take away that stress." It would be funny if it weren't so true.

I feel the tears well up again, but try to subtly wipe them away.

"What do the tears mean?" Dr. Miller asks, gently prodding me to notice my own feelings. There's no hiding from her.

"I think I feel like there's no way to fix the reasons why I'm sinking. Because I can't fix COVID or the overwhelming feeling of being a psychiatrist during COVID. I keep wondering if maybe my level of exhaustion is just a physical manifestation of the state of our mental health system. As my clinic fills up and the people I see seem sicker, I'm also feeling worse than usual—tired, forgetful, and disconnected. My grandmother says I'm everyone's substitute teddy bear right now, but sometimes I feel more like an emotional sponge, or even a punching bag."

"I hear you. . . . I feel all that, too, if it helps to know that."

It does. As I respect her immensely, when she admits that she struggles with things in her job, especially the same things as me, I instantly feel less alone.

"Well, I'm not glad you feel like that, obviously, but yes, it does help to know. What I'm noticing, too, is that every conversation with a patient or a friend is a version of the same thing. I listen to the same problems day in and day out, which also happen to be a lot of my own problems, or my friends' problems, or a family member's problems. It feels a lot harder to distance myself from what I'm hearing, which makes it hard for me to put my head down and focus on my job."

Dr. Miller looks back, nodding slightly. "It's a lot harder to not experience feelings about a patient—countertransference, if you want to call it that—when you're actively experiencing a lot of the same struggles."

"It's never-ending, that's how it feels right now, like the week of a mass shooting, when everyone is talking about it in appointments, and people are talking about it around me socially, too. I'll come home emotionally exhausted afterwards—so much so that I don't want to talk to anyone or watch the news. One story of trauma is enough, but a whole day's worth? There's no room to breathe."

"In moments like this, it's really hard to be a therapist, but no one talks about that," she agrees. Again, I feel a rush of appreciation that she is being so open with me about her own struggles. "Plus," she continues, "I also wonder if you're feeling more vulnerable now because you're also experiencing all the other things we've talked about—feeling lonely sometimes, and not sleeping, and being so tired. Those things make it even harder to put up that necessary barrier between doctor and patient."

"Oh, my God, yes! The more exhausted I feel, the harder it is to remove myself. It's like I can't protect myself anymore. I remember when I found out that my dog was dying during my residency. He'd been with me all through college, then medical school and after, and when he was suddenly sick and not getting better, I struggled to work." The feelings from the time flood back to me as I remember going numb and not quite being present with patients. The longer he was in the animal hospital, and the less sleep I got, the harder it was to distance myself from their stories—from anything, really. Suddenly, the world at work, which is a pretty dark world, pierced through my everyday life, and I was more or less aware of that darkness constantly.

I continue speaking through deep breaths and a few tears. "It's like somebody turned up the volume on the background noise of patients' traumas. I remember crying about something a patient experienced after they left my office. It surprised me at the time. I don't really break like that . . ."

"It's a lot harder to remain distant when you are struggling yourself," Dr. Miller summarizes.

"Yes, especially if it seems like *no one* is really improving."

She blinks, and I can tell I've struck a nerve. "Is your job," she asks, "to only help people get better?"

"What do you mean?"

"Well, don't you think there's more to your job than fixing people?"

I start to reflect on the benefits I've experienced from having Dr. Miller in my life, and I understand what she means. Simply having someone who is there and listening helps healing. And yet, I think there is something different as a psychiatrist. The medical model emphasizes medications and treatments to improve symptoms and quality of life in a patient. To *fix* them. When that's not happening, it's hard not to feel like I'm failing at my job. I just wasn't taught to see the other benefits in what I do.

I reply somewhat tangentially, "One of the hardest things is that when people *do* get better, they stop coming to see me. I was taught that my job is to make people well enough so that they don't need to see me, but that leaves me with a caseload of suffering people who aren't getting better or new people who are also acutely suffering. Maybe it's the nature of psychiatry or the pandemic, but it really starts to feel as if no one is doing well. That's overwhelming."

"It could also be because you see college kids and healthcare workers and their families and those groups, especially, are really struggling right now," Dr. Miller offers. "I will tell you that I have seen people get better, even now, if that helps."

"It does." I smile a bit. "I just know that I get a lot of meaning when I see treatment work, so I feel really ineffective in my job right now. It's all kind of a recipe for disaster. Honestly, I wish I could tell the people who are better that I want to see them more, because it makes *me* feel better. I saw a patient the other day who is easy and stable, and she just needed to check in. She actually apologized to me, saying, 'I must be SO boring for you.' And, I was like, 'No! Come back all the time! You're doing well and I don't see that enough.' I meant it, but obviously that's not a thing."

I laugh, and Dr. Miller does, too, before I go on. "Something I've been thinking about, and struggling with, too, is when I look forward into the future, I know that for people like us, for mental health providers, this doesn't just end with COVID. I think maybe things will get even worse when people can finally breathe and stop running on adrenaline, and have time to think about everything that has happened and how much their mental health has been affected. I keep telling that to media people who interview me, but it's such a Debbie Downer answer."

Dr. Miller looks at me a bit seriously. "It's a real one, though. Can I ask you a question?"

"Sure."

"Has healthcare, or mental health care specifically, ever in your lifetime, *not* been broken, or at least imperfect? Like, have the people who needed to see you gotten in for an appointment quickly, or even afforded their treatments?"

"Well, of course not," I say, recognizing that clearly all of what's going on now is really just an exacerbation of the problems that have always made the field challenging, like lack of access to mental health care. And maybe some cognitive distortions of overgeneralizing and catastrophizing on my part.

"So, why expect it to change now?" she asks, reasonably. "It's just . . . another time . . . when it is *still* bad and we just have to adapt to it."

"You're right. I need to start looking at things like that. Instead of like doomsday."

"Yes! And, it's also why you need to think more about having rituals between patients as a way to leave one person's story behind, before going to the next. And a ritual for the end of the day. So you won't carry patients with you."

We've had this conversation a few times, but I haven't done much to change my behavior. Dr. Miller has suggested I try doing stretches after work or even walk around my kitchen between patients, but I only do it sometimes. I understand her suggestion, but when it comes down to it, I'm too tired to change anything and don't seem to have the minutes to spare. Just like so many of my patients.

"I knooooow," I say, leaning back on the couch. "You mean, peeing in between visits isn't enough?" After spending the vast majority of medical school and residency not acknowledging my needs, including eating and urination, just getting to the bathroom feels like a step in the right direction. And, I'm a psychiatrist. Ask a surgeon if *they* take care of their needs.

Dr. Miller laughs, "Well, peeing is important, but no. I mean, a ritual that is more centered and mindful. Even in the realm of some of the *woo woo* stuff you get mad at me for suggesting."

I do hate the *woo woo*. I'm far too sarcastic and cynical for most of it (like meditation or crystals), and it can feel anything but relaxing to me.

"Okay, let's try this," she says, undeterred. "You know Mr. Rogers? Remember how he would enter a room?"

I start to sing the "Won't You Be My Neighbor" song in my head and say, "Yes! I love him."

"So, you know how he had that transition where he'd walk to the closet, take off his jacket, and hang it up?" I nod.

"And then he'd put on his sweater and change his shoes?" I nod again.

"You need something like that, to metaphorically take off your jacket before the next person and leave whatever is going on in their lives with them, so all the sad stories don't just accumulate."

"That makes sense. Taking off the jacket of people's problems."

I know I have to try.

———

I try to get back into a groove and find my confidence again, but it's not just patients I am faltering with. Sitting at home, lounging around after work, I get a calendar alert on my phone that says, simply, "meeting." I have no idea what it's about, but it's due to happen in thirty minutes. *Really helpful, Jessi*, I mutter to myself judgmentally.

Anxious, I start to search for an email, a note, or really anything that points to whom I'm supposed to meet with. Owing to my serious overcommitment habit, it really could be anything—a meeting with HR to discuss the administrative work I've been doing to support faculty and staff mental health. Or, maybe I'm supposed to give a talk about our mental health resources to a specific department, or even give a national talk on burnout among healthcare workers. All these things happen multiple times a week, in addition to my seeing patients. As Dr. Miller reminds me, these "extracurricular activities" take a toll on me.

Just as I've resigned myself to the fact that someone, somewhere, is about to be angry or feel let down by my non-appearance, I get an email saying, "Dr. Gold, are you logging into the Zoom soon?"

I can feel my heart drop into my stomach as I sit in front of my computer, eating a sandwich, in a hoodie (of course). Basically, the classic example of *no, not at all ready to log into Zoom.*

I look up the sender's email address and notice that it's from an organization I vaguely remember promising to give a talk for. "That's TODAY?" I internally scream. The screen starts to blur as I now realize an entire group of people are waiting for me to give an actual presentation, one that is supposed to start momentarily. The worst-case scenario.

I put my sandwich down and start scrolling my email to figure out what my talk is even supposed to be about. I come to: *Coping with COVID While Taking Care of Ourselves.*

The irony is not lost on me that I am so distracted and exhausted that I forgot I was giving a talk on how to prevent these very symptoms, though I almost napped through another similar presentation last week. I woke up two minutes before it. I should have learned my lesson then.

Suddenly, I remember that I gave a talk a few months ago with almost the same name as today's supposed talk. It was called *How Are You Really? Coping with COVID While Taking Care of Ourselves.* I decide it can be repurposed, mostly because I have no choice. So, I make a new title slide in one minute and save it as today's date.

I then allow myself another minute to run upstairs and put on a nice top, over an actual bra. I keep my sweatpants on, but going braless in a T-shirt in front of fifty people would cross a line. I run back downstairs, out of breath, and open the link in the reminder email. I look down at the clock on my computer and see that I'm only about five minutes late. *That was pretty fast*, I think to myself with pride. The pride quickly fades when I open the meeting and see all the people waiting for me.

To save face, before I introduce myself, I start with what this group probably suspects is a white lie. "Sorry about that; I had trouble logging in." The easy excuse for all things right now. I lie because I am embarrassed and upset, but also because I can't say to them what I couldn't admit to myself. As with James, my forgotten patient, the real problem is me.

The only person with their camera turned on nods, and I imagine everyone else I can't see is judging me. That's what those little black squares let me do: imagine the worst. I grew up in a family where we always arrived at a concert or show early, waiting quietly in our seats as everyone else filed in at the last minute, just as the lights were dimming. And I've taken that to heart. My friends, and therapist, know that I'll text if I'm going to be late by even a single minute. I value punctuality.

I'm also a person who typically gets a lot of things done, often at the same time. I've been asked repeatedly how I do it all, and I don't have a great answer other than that I've always done things this way, without a problem. Supervisors have been concerned with how much I'm putting on my plate. In residency, my program director and mentor regularly told me I was doing too much and would burn out. I laughed, told her I liked it all, and assured her I'd be fine. Somehow, I *was* fine. But I'm not fine anymore. My ability to juggle has turned into a lot of balls dropping at once.

I feel like I now have every symptom of ADHD (attention deficit hyperactivity disorder) that I screen my patients for, including being easily distracted, having trouble prioritizing tasks, and feeling forgetful (um, case in point; see also: James). With all the changes to work and school during the pandemic, not to mention random work-from-home distractions like leaf blowers and barking dogs, it's no wonder I'm seeing so many patients who complain of feeling distracted right now. In fact, having trouble concentrating is the second most common complaint I'm seeing in my office. The first, incidentally, is exhaustion.

As I tell patients, concentration is a tough symptom to nail down because it can be affected by anxiety, depression, trauma, burnout, substance use, and lack of sleep. It's really hard to know the root cause; often, it's a combination of the above. For me, though, it's probably caused by whatever is making me so damn tired all the time.

Just thinking about it all makes me even more worried about whatever is going on with me than I have been before. Forgetting that I committed to giving a talk—something that could affect my professional reputation—is more than a warning. It's a big red flashing danger sign.

16

"I'M STILL NOT working, and the guilt is pretty much eating at me," Luke admits, looking slightly more relaxed than he sounds in a T-shirt and jeans at home. If I'm calculating correctly, he has been on leave from work for four or five weeks. In medical residency terms, that's a lifetime. "I guess there *is* something new to tell you, though. Instead of only worrying about being infected by COVID, I now have obsessive thoughts about what people are thinking about me, or wondering about me, or assuming about me because of my recent life changes, especially my co-residents who have had to cover for me for *soooooo* long now."

"It's hard not to wonder what they might be thinking," I affirm. "Did you tell anyone the truth about why you're out?"

"No," he says, looking somewhat ashamed. "I mean, my boyfriend obviously knows, and my family knows, and you and my therapist know, but my co-residents were just told that I had a personal emergency. It was all kept pretty vague. The way I wanted it."

My immediate impulse is to ask him why he hasn't told his colleagues and wider circle of friends the truth, but my wiser mind tells me to wait. I don't want to jump right into that topic and risk making him feel judged. Instead, I try shaping the conversation so he is apt to lead me toward the answer I'm seeking. "I wonder, what would you think about someone in your position if you were the one covering for a co-resident for unknown reasons?" In this, I'm playing the classic, *Think about how you would talk to a good friend* move, a version of what I told Megan to use to help her with her automatic negative thoughts about herself.

"I've actually thought about that when I can't sleep at night. If I were them, I'd probably be okay covering for a day or two, and respect that they had to make that choice. I wouldn't even question the reason." I nod, hoping he hears himself saying this. "But having to change schedules for months to cover for someone would irk me, to say the least. To be honest, I'd also probably be digging for gossip to find out what was wrong." He pauses and adds, "I'd also hope they were okay because I'm not a completely *horrible* person."

I smile at Luke, feeling warmth for him. "I know you're not a horrible person. And what are you worried they're saying and thinking about *you*?"

"To be honest, I think they'll assume that given my prolonged absence, I'm not cut out for medicine. That something is wrong with me."

Luke's answer doesn't surprise me. These kinds of fears are why many health professionals don't get help, or hide it when they do, and prompt me to think about how much I hate gossip and the impact it can have on people's self-esteem.

What I want to know now is what lies beneath Luke's concerns. "Do you think those things about yourself?" I gently prod him.

"Probably." He pauses for a heartbeat. "*Damn*. Yes, I totally do. Especially because right now, I'm not able to do something I've always dreamed of doing—practice medicine. So, by definition, I've failed."

This hits close to home. "I don't know if this helps, but I don't think you've failed," I tell Luke, attempting to validate his experience and also reassure him I believe he's doing the right thing by taking a break from work to get help. "I think there is a reframe here you could try—that instead of failing in your job, you're focused on getting better, which over time will make you better able to do your job and make you a better, more empathetic doctor and leader. It may not be how you're used to viewing a situation like the one you are in—and the fact that you're in the middle of it makes it doubly hard—I realize that."

"Thanks, I hope you're right, Dr. Gold, about my getting better. I'm just afraid I won't be able to go back to work at all. Could that actually happen?"

"I don't like to make predictions because mental health is truly unpredictable. I also don't want to lie to you. Being a resident is a hard thing in the first place, and being a resident in a pandemic—especially when you have a consuming fear of being infected with COVID—is especially hard. You're not in a position to do on-the-job exposure therapy, because you can't go to work gradually, exposing yourself to potentially germ-filled situations bit by bit. As a resident, you also can't control your schedule at your hospital like that. It's an all-or-nothing situation—you're either back or you're not. So, realistically, that could make it hard to return to work any time soon. On the other hand, you might continue to get better and feel well enough to go back and be fine. I wish I knew."

"I appreciate your honesty. I just really hope I can go back. I can't imagine doing anything else."

"I hope so, too. I'm not sure if this helps," I try, "but it might make sense to at least start to conceptualize your OCD as a chronic illness— one that might not ever really go away, even if you get back to work."

"I'm trying to come to terms with that. In therapy, I've become pretty good at noticing which thoughts are just my OCD acting up, and I'll pause, label them as that, and then let them be."

"I think that's a good sign that therapy is working," I say emphatically.

"I do too, but one thing that makes it harder for me to accept is that all anyone talks about when it comes to mental health is depression or anxiety. Somehow, people understand those disorders and accept them, and they've become almost normal. But, no one talks about OCD, or schizophrenia, or bipolar, for that matter. At least in medicine."

My curiosity is piqued. "I've never thought of that distinction. What made you start thinking about that?"

"Well, a lot of things, I guess. Like during Mental Health Awareness month, the stories in the media always seem to say, 'I was depressed or anxious and now I'm better.' In other words, most are about people who have some kind of relatively 'acceptable' mental illness and then get over it." He takes a deep breath.

"And what they're saying is, 'I'm stable now, so don't worry about me, I'm qualified to do whatever I do.' The thing is, *my* mental illness will probably never be completely in the past. It will always be there, a low-lying hum of obsessions. In that context, I can see why someone might not know what to think of my OCD diagnosis, especially because I'm a doctor. I'm not supposed to be sick."

"Is that why you haven't told many people the reason you're out?"

"Maybe. I guess I worry that if I tell people what's going on with me, everything I do from now on will be seen through the lens of my having a mental illness."

"What do you mean 'seen through a lens of having mental illness'?" I repeat his words back to him to clarify what he is feeling.

Luke explains, "It's like I can't just be mad, or tired anymore. If I'm having a bad day, people might think, *Oh, is that his OCD?*"

As someone who has stayed up writing until 2 a.m. because I'm in a groove, I can attest that certain behaviors, even if they seem like symptoms of an illness like hypomania, aren't diagnoses. To Luke, I say, "The way I see it, you can be tired, you can be sad, you may even drink too much one night, and all of it might affect your demeanor at work or socially. But that doesn't mean any of those things have anything to do with your OCD."

"We're just humans," he says. The two of us share a look of understanding.

Luke continues, "Another reason I'm not telling anyone is I know they'll try to give me advice or even treat me—I honestly hate it when someone says something ridiculous like 'Have you considered talking to a therapist?' I want to tell them, 'That ship has sailed, honey. I go three times a week.' Plus, there's a layer of shame in it all. I think we use 'you should go to therapy' as a way of saying someone needs fixing, or as punishment for bad behavior."

"Oh yeah, the bad boyfriend, or toxic friend, or erratic celebrity who should 'just go to therapy.'"

Luke laughs and I think about how therapists and psychiatrists talk a good game about the importance of going to therapy to help them in the work they do. But if someone *needs* to go for themselves, for personal reasons, that's another story.

To Luke, I say, "I'm hopeful that, with time, you'll feel that taking the risk and getting help was the right thing. No matter what ends up happening with work. I mean, *I'm* proud of you for asking for help, if that matters." I always feel good when I get a pat on the back from my therapist, so I try to spread the love. Plus, I am actually proud of him and hope he knows I'm on his team, no matter if he is a doctor again soon or not. Though, I have hope he will be and he's headed in the right direction.

"It does help," he says softly.

I add, pointedly, "I know it's difficult, but do your best to take things one day at a time. You can start by telling one person you trust, maybe someone who isn't even a resident with you, and maybe you don't even tell them everything. You simply start the conversation, and see how people, including you, feel about it and react. Do you think you could tell at least one person in the next few weeks? It might help settle all the thoughts swirling in your head."

"I can try."

"The serenity prayer may also be helpful to you. You know, 'God grant me the serenity to accept the things I cannot change, the courage to change the things I can, and the wisdom to know the difference.' You might have heard about it from people in recovery or AA, or even those with other serious chronic illness, but it really is a helpful mentality for most of us. It doesn't have to be to God, though, and can just be some higher power instead. It's just about acknowledging that some things are bigger than us and out of our control. Especially recently, a lot of patients have really found solace in it as a philosophy of life. There is really nothing more out of our control than a global pandemic. For you, it can help you focus on the things you can change, like getting more support, rather than on the things you can't, like having OCD and needing to be off work right now."

Luke sighs audibly. "I think I'm still working on the part about the wisdom to know the difference."

"Aren't we all?"

My session with Luke reminds me of my own experiences about what it means to be on antidepressants: It wasn't until recently that I realized it was something I was ashamed of.

I was first diagnosed with depression in college, and pretty quickly I agreed to take a medication, Wellbutrin, which happened to work well, and my symptoms got better. I wasn't sleeping as much during the day, I was more motivated, and I stopped feeling so down. If I were a psychiatrist seeing me, I'd call me an easy patient. My first and only med worked, and it worked quickly.

Aside from a few blips here and there, I've been stable for about fourteen years.

But even though I essentially spend all day prescribing medication and telling people that taking a prescription for mental health reasons is just like taking meds for heart disease or diabetes, I've never talked publicly about my being on medication. To be fair, maybe it's always weird to tell colleagues about one's mental health history and psychiatric medications. But, I've managed to be open and honest about many of my mental health struggles—that I go to therapy regularly, that I've struggled through the pandemic, and some of the tips and tricks I've learned from Dr. Miller—and still, when it comes to taking an antidepressant, something has been stopping me from telling. Something feels different.

I wasn't cognitively aware of my hesitancy until an X conversation I had in July 2020. It was only three months ago, but it feels like years—COVID months being more like years, or dog years, at this point.

I remember scrolling and coming across a post from an ER physician with a large social media following, in which she discussed her own mental health and the stigma of any medical professional seeking help. Her words went viral, as did many of the responses from healthcare workers that followed. I read all of them, knowing I was reading something special, because of its rarity.

"I'm a pediatric oncologist/palliative care doctor. I'm a recovering alcoholic with a history of depression/suicidal ideation. Mental health treatment saved my life."

"I'm an ER/ICU RN and I couldn't give patients the care they need or support my co-workers if I didn't see a therapist weekly."

"I'm a psychiatrist. This Tweet is the first time I have publicly shared that I have seen a therapist."

Almost without thinking about it, I found myself tweeting: "I'm a psychiatrist. If I didn't see a therapist, I wouldn't be able to see healthcare workers as patients because I wouldn't be healthy enough to help." Maybe it was the pandemic, but for the first time ever, it felt as if change was happening. Or, maybe it was just that everyone in medicine had reached their breaking point and simply couldn't hold it in anymore.

We all know from watching celebrities who talk about their mental health struggles that sometimes all it takes is for one person to open up; that starts a domino effect of opening up and self-disclosure. The stories from healthcare workers I was reading on X felt similarly cathartic—like a backed-up dam was bursting.

Except when I look back on my tweet now, I realize it was incomplete. Unlike so many of the others, I hadn't admitted to being on medication. Despite prescribing medications and believing in the power of medications, I left out that part of my story.

Did I do it intentionally? I wondered that night, unable to sleep, staring at the ceiling, then at my phone. *Why didn't I mention medication in that tweet?* I asked myself over and over again. It was like counting identical thoughts, instead of sheep.

The next day, each time I typed an order for a prescription, the thought arose again, unbidden: *Am I stigmatizing medication by not talking about my own experience?*

My incomplete story makes me feel inauthentic and, worse, like a hypocrite. Because I *believe* in these medications. I also encourage vulnerability in others and praise their public self-disclosures. If I can't talk about my own medication, how can I tell patients to feel okay about their choice to take medication? And there it is: Being a mental health practitioner doesn't protect me from the stigma. If my hesitation is still so strong, what does that mean for everyone else?

At the same time, I realize I don't owe anyone every detail of my story. I get to choose what parts of my medical history I care to share, or not share any of it. Making myself vulnerable in that way could be powerful and help people. But admitting that I've been taking a psychotropic medication for more than a decade still feels like a line I am not ready to cross.

At my next session with Dr. Miller, I tell her about my dilemma. Her response: "Okay, but do you even want to be public about it?" Like any good therapist, she is keeping my best interests at heart.

"Good question," I say. *And one I'd ask my own patients*, I think. "I'm starting to believe that I *need* to."

"*Need* to?" she echoes.

"Yes, for authenticity's sake. I feel like a fake telling people to take meds and that meds are fine and not to worry, but acting differently when it's about me and my history."

"You don't need to tell anyone anything. You can be authentic and not tell your story to patients."

"Yeah, I know. But that doesn't feel like the authenticity I *want*. There are things I might never be willing to say publicly, but I feel like I should be able to talk about *this*. It's not traumatic, and I've been on Wellbutrin for *years* at this point. I want to at least understand why I haven't talked about it or why it feels like I can't."

She then asks me something I find myself asking so many of my patients who question being on medication. "What does being on medication mean to you?"

"My first gut answer is that it means I'm sicker."

"Sicker?"

"Yeah, like if you need meds, if you need to see a psychiatrist versus just needing therapy alone, you are worse off. That's me. Worse off."

"What does being 'worse off' mean?"

"Well, that I'm different, or permanently broken in some way." *Broken* is such a heavy word and, as I say it out loud, I feel simultaneously ashamed, shocked, and angry. I had no idea I thought this, despite my years of therapy. I find myself starting to wonder how my formerly buried beliefs have been impacting me and whether, even if they're unconscious, they might affect my patient care.

Dr. Miller can tell that my mind is going; she knows me well. "That's a powerful thing to acknowledge," she says. "What would it mean, then, if someone else knew?"

"That I'm a bad doctor in some way." I pause, hearing myself say out loud what I've fought against my patients believing—something I've publicly advocated to change. "Whoa, that's fucked up."

"What is?"

"That I said that. I mean clearly I must believe it somewhere in my soul if I said it. But I also go around telling people it's not true and I believe that, too. I don't think I'm lying to them, but there's clearly a disconnect."

"I can see why that might feel distressing. I want to tell you something that I've never told a patient. Can I tell you?" She shifts a little in her seat, maybe suggesting some anxiety is associated with what she wants to say.

"Always."

"So, I take medication, the same one as you, and have for a while." She shifts again slightly and takes a deep breath. "Does that change your opinion of me?"

Without pausing or thinking, because I don't need to, I reply, "Oh, gosh, no, it could never." I finish the trail of my thoughts in my head. *You're pretty past reproach at this point. You're the best therapist I've ever had.* I don't say this out loud in case she thinks the praise is creepy.

She continues, to really drive her point home, "So, why would anyone view *you* differently?"

I'm a bit blown away by the power of her revelation to make me see something I couldn't quite see before. Kind of like when I ask patients to think about how they'd react to a friend telling them something potentially upsetting, only Dr. Miller isn't a friend. She's a fellow professional, which makes her revelation even more powerful.

What I say out loud is, "If anything, what you told me makes me trust you more."

Dr. Miller smiles. "Exactly."

17

_____

DESPITE THE BREAKTHROUGHS I've been having in therapy, I still feel as if I'm hanging on by a thread. Last night, I had to set three alarms to make sure I woke up for work—at 6:10, 6:15, and 6:20; otherwise I wouldn't be motivated to get out of bed. I feel the way some patients have told me they feel when they take sleep medication for insomnia— as if they have a hangover without ever having a drink. I guess that means I have a life hangover. Maybe it's a sign.

On some level, I know I can do better than allotting a single hour a week to take care of myself—my Thursday sessions with Dr. Miller. For one thing, it's better to have more than one formal source of support (outside of friends and family) to help me deal. After all, I wouldn't want patients relying solely on me to cope. Clearly, I need to reframe self-care as not being selfish, or a waste of my time. *I can put me first and still be a good friend and a good psychiatrist*, I keep telling myself.

The first thing I try picking up again is journaling, even if a part of me thinks it's a little silly. *I already like to write*, I tell myself, *so at least it will be easy.* Dr. Miller suggested it a few months back, but I never got into it. I was never a kid who wrote consistently in diaries, and the few I have from my childhood are half filled, consisting mainly of complaints about being teased by my brother or having had a fight with a friend. When I look back on them, I notice that the common theme is rage. That's also the theme of my last journal entry from when Dr. Miller initially suggested it. I'd written about a patient calling multiple times despite my being busy in clinic with no time to call back during the work day. "I have no time or energy for this shit, and I hate every minute of it" is what I wrote. It seems I only really want to write in a journal when I'm pissed off—so, maybe I should call it a rage journal. Dr. Miller says that's okay, as long as it helps.

I grab a pink gel pen and prop open up my small black and purple notebook with the Taylor Swift lyrics "She had a marvelous time ruining everything" printed on the cover, and I start to write. I have to admit that pouring things out on paper without worrying about syntax, or grammar, or even meaning can feel like a relief. Sometimes, I even catch myself thinking about how these little rage snippets could become the basis of articles, which Dr. Miller has repeatedly told me is not the point. That's why I've started journaling with paper and pen, rather than on a computer. If I feel the urge to turn a journal entry into something publishable, I have to take a lot more steps to make it happen. That increases the chances I'll keep my journaling private and only for me, like it's supposed to be.

I'm so used to writing on a computer, or even on my phone, that holding a pen feels weird at first, but it becomes easier as I keep writing. Muscle memory, I guess. I set a goal to write for around fifteen minutes, since the data on journaling suggest that's the length of time it takes to accrue mental health benefits.[1] I don't set an alarm, though, because that will make the whole thing feel stressful, like taking an exam.

As I write, I catch my mind wandering away to a song I heard on TikTok, or a news story I read. But for the most part, I'm just focused on my rage. Mostly, I'm angry at myself: *Why can't I just suck it up and work through my fatigue?*

Afterward, I actually do feel some minor relief. I've put in my daily quota of *me time,* and I make a plan to do it every day for the rest of the week. When I fail to follow through with that goal, I sign myself up for a (virtual) weekend retreat that's billed as a combination of meditation and breathwork training. Even though I'm personally averse to mindfulness, which is what this clearly is, and I have gone to great lengths to avoid it (like telling my entire residency class I didn't want to start our mandatory process groups—group therapy with each other—with five minutes of it, and saying I'd come late, instead—only to be told it's everyone or no one; my position made it no one), I know I need to take drastic measures. But between the gongs and the timed inhalations and exhalations, and the earnest faces as the person in my class says they "saw colors," I end up feeling ridiculous, not healed.

Mindfulness just isn't the answer for me. Don't get me wrong; it definitely is for someone. But I need to find another coping skill of choice. I know I should try to think about it more, as I tell my patients, like finding a hobby—something I will actually do and enjoy, and not a one-size-fits-all solution. But it's hard. I need to remember that just because the hospital promotes or funds mindfulness, that doesn't mean it's the only solution or, if I hate it (which I do), I'm somehow "bad at coping" (something, unfortunately, I've heard from many of my patients about the prescribed coping skills).

When I tell Dr. Miller about my efforts, she actually laughs. "Of course, you hated it," she says. "You did a full weekend of mindfulness when you can barely handle ten minutes!"

I wanted to defend myself and tell her that sometimes, people do illogical things, especially when they feel helpless, and especially when their patients and the evidence[2] suggest it is effective. Instead, I let it go, and turn to a method I have always trusted. Like any good person in medicine (with the added benefit of having doctors in the family), I make an appointment to see my primary care physician.

I'm convinced there must be a medical reason I feel so tired.

———

Dr. Fredrickson is younger than I am, and newly out of residency. I've seen him around the hospital, and I've got the impression he is thorough and deliberate.

When we hop onto a Zoom appointment, I tell him I'm so tired I can barely function, and he proceeds to get a full history of my chief complaint, or "presenting problem," as we are taught to do in medical school. "How long has your fatigue been going on?" Months. "How much is it affecting your day-to-day life?" Significantly. "What's your sleep like?" Horrible, because of all my impromptu naps. He asks about my other symptoms (lack of concentration) and medications (Wellbutrin). He double-checks that my alcohol use hasn't increased. It hasn't. I am one of the rare people who seem to be drinking less than before the pandemic.

Then, after ruling out physical problems, he gets to the heart of it, and asks, "What's your mood like?" which makes me smile. I'm glad he has asked me this question because he should. Many patients with mood issues see only a primary care doctor, and if they don't screen for or recognize a patient's mental health needs, that person often goes undiagnosed and untreated, which can be dangerous. People who die by suicide often visit their doctor in the month before they die, and for 45 percent, that doctor is a primary care provider; only 20 percent see a mental health professional.[3] In other words, primary care is often the first, and only defense—which is why routine mental health screening is critical.

Even though I'm a psychiatrist myself, I've never actually seen a psychiatrist to manage my medication. That may seem odd, given what I do, but I have told myself I don't need to because my symptoms haven't gotten worse. Primary care has always handled my Wellbutrin.

I nod at my doctor. "I appreciate you asking that question. Truthfully, my mood has been normal. I mean, I'm definitely busy with work and that's hard, and I'm lonely without seeing people all of the time, but I'm also not sad."

Dr. Fredrickson does not look convinced. "Are you interested in things that you usually like to do?"

"Yeah, but I can't do a lot of them because most things are canceled or closed. Like I have a shirt that says, 'I miss concerts and hugs,' and I mean it. I do."

His face is still stern as he asks, "And any thoughts of suicide?"

"No." I pause and notice I'm feeling defensive. "I also see a therapist weekly."

He nods and takes a deep breath. I'm fidgeting in the silence, so I continue. "I feel like maybe you don't believe me that I'm not depressed. I promise you, I'm not. I'm aware of what depression feels like, and this isn't it. I just *know* that the cause of my fatigue is something physical, not mental."

In that moment, I understand exactly how so many of my patients feel when someone sees *anxiety* or *depression* on their chart and assumes that's the cause of all their complaints. I find myself feeling agitated for all of us. I've heard story after story of serious diagnoses like heart attacks or infectious diseases being missed because doctors have focused on what they assume is the most glaring issue and miss the true cause of the problem. I've also seen it from the other side, as a psychiatrist, when a patient of mine in inpatient psychiatry, who had schizophrenia, was sent to our inpatient psychiatric ward from the emergency room after episodes of what they called "psychogenic vomiting" (a.k.a. vomiting that isn't caused by any physical problem). But when our psychiatric team actually palpated his stomach, we discovered masses—and ultimately had confirmation with the finally ordered scans; the patient had cancer everywhere. The doctors who first evaluated him just attributed all his symptoms to his schizophrenia and dismissed him to psychiatry.

This bias is also seen in the literature: in a study of 300 family physicians in Iowa, physicians were less likely to believe that a patient with abdominal pain or a headache had a serious illness if they had a previous history of depression, compared to patients with no past history; they were also less likely to order testing for the patient.[4] In this context, it is perhaps less surprising, but no less shocking, that people with schizophrenia and other severe mental illnesses have a reduced life expectancy compared to the general population. This is often caused by other comorbid physical health problems, like heart disease or diabetes, rather than the mental illness itself.[5]

Maybe Dr. Fredrickson can tell I'm getting angry, because he asks, kindly, "What are *you* thinking is going on?"

"I don't know exactly, but I can tell you that when I'm tired, my body feels extremely heavy, but not like the exhaustion that comes with depression. I don't know how to explain it, but it isn't at all related to my mood. I fall asleep without meaning to and fight to stay awake while seeing patients. That's not okay or normal for me. Also, caffeine doesn't help."

I take a deep breath and continue, noticing my speech is rather fast, as if I'm trying to convince him before he breaks in. "I feel like I need labs at least, to test for whatever could be making me have low energy, like my thyroid or iron or B_{12}?"

"We can do that and see what it shows," he says, but to my eyes, he still seems unconvinced. "I don't have a problem ordering labs," he continues. "It's just . . ." He pauses. "I hope you will also let me know if you think your mood is off and you need an adjustment in your meds."

"I will," I say, telling myself that he is just being careful but feeling defensive anyway. For good measure, I add, "I just want you to know that I mainly see healthcare workers, and I get why we're stoic and afraid to get help, and how hard it is, but if I needed help, I'd ask for it. I have before and I will again. Plus, I'm a psychiatrist, so I *hope* I'd believe in the brain-body connection and that depression can be a cause of physical symptoms."

He smiles, finally, then orders my bloodwork. I may not have convinced him, but at least I got what I wanted. Many of my patients aren't that lucky.

After my appointment, I go to the lab for a blood test, and as I wait my turn, I flash back to when I was learning to draw blood as a medical student, a memory that comes up pretty much every time I have bloodwork done. As students, we did many blood draws on each other, along with other procedures, starting with the physical exam, which meant looking up each other's noses and in each other's ears, before we progressed to the more invasive sticking-each-other-with-a-needle phase. When it was my turn to try to draw blood in our learning exercise, I was the last to attempt on one of my classmates who was a bodybuilder with great veins (and thus the group pincushion). Despite the supervising nurse telling me I should have learned from the others before me and so, *clearly* I would be perfect and we could leave, I missed twice, and she threatened to fail me. That only worsened my anxiety, so I missed again. I started to cry, and all the nurses and my classmates gathered around me, which is pretty much my worst nightmare. Luckily, the fourth needle stick was the charm.

I still remember my relief as I was finally leaving the room, high-fiving my classmate as he put yet another Band-Aid on his arm. When a nurse asked me what specialty I wanted to go into, I was even able to jokingly retort: "Something nonprocedural, I'll tell you that!" The remaining nurses and students laughed loudly. They may have thought I was kidding, but I knew then and there that I was much better with words than with needles.

A few days later, I got a phone notification that my blood test results were ready on the MyChart app, a system that anyone who has seen a physician in a major teaching hospital is all too familiar with. These days, patients not only can see their labs but often are able to see them before their doctors do, which is not always a great thing. I've heard stories of people seeing positive cancer pathology reports before anyone has told them they have cancer. I wish people would wait, but the temptation is hard to ignore.

I glance at my various numbers and start making interpretations, trying to remember what I learned in my internal medicine rotations in residency. My thyroid and iron levels are normal, but my B_{12} is flagged as low: normal is 232 to 1345, and mine is 211. Low B_{12} can also cause depression, so it's one of the most common labs ordered by a psychiatrist. I'm familiar enough with it that after seeing my results, I felt confident that my doctor will put me on a B_{12} supplement of some kind. Sure enough, within a few hours, Dr. Fredrickson calls and says he wants to start me on B_{12} injections, once a week for about a month, until my numbers get back up. I excitedly agree, feeling relieved—and vindicated. *It's a physical health problem, after all.*

A few injections, and my energy would be back to normal. Or, so I very strongly wish.

18

"HI, SORRY, I didn't have time to change, I came right from doing mock medical school interviews with the premed advisors." Naya is breathing a bit heavily, which suggests she probably ran back to her dorm room for this telehealth visit. Though she's back on campus, she still mostly spends her time studying and taking classes in her dorm room, along with social distancing, testing, and masking. But at least she isn't stuck at home anymore, which many of my college student patients describe as being "on pause" from the traditional version of college (and their expected one). They are just waiting for someone to finally hit play again.

Naya is dressed in a suit, and wearing another beautiful pair of earrings, this time with turquoise stones. I try to think of the last time I wore a suit—probably when I was interviewing for my residency. It's hard to imagine under what circumstances I'd get that dressed up now. I quickly reply, "I don't care what you wear—I'm struggling to do more than just put on a work-appropriate top, if that helps." I shift the computer view so she can see my sweatpants. She laughs.

I look forward to seeing Naya. Maybe because I self-disclosed a bit last time about my own experiences taking tests as a premed and medical student, I feel I can be more real with her. Or maybe, I just organically really like her. Whatever the reason, I feel a little bit lighter talking to her than I have the rest of today. It's needed and nice. "So, how'd the mock interviews go?" I ask, hesitantly, not wanting to change the tone of the conversation but knowing I need to ask.

"Ugh. I don't think the advisors like me. Or, maybe they think I can't get in so I'm not worth their time."

"Did they say that?" I am trying to help her distinguish what is said versus what's assumed, as my therapist so often does for me.

"Well, no one said that explicitly, but when they asked me about my scores, I told them about my anxiety, which was a factor, and that it was something I was actively working on. I felt good about that, about owning my stuff and being truthful, but instantly, I could tell I'd said the wrong thing."

"What told you that?"

"They shot each other these looks, then changed the subject— no validation or thank you for sharing, nothing."

As she says this, I think about how often people bravely expose their struggles to someone who isn't able to support them, or worse, harbors significant bias or stigma. The way someone reacts when we reveal a difficult truth ("Were you drinking?" "Did you say no?" "Are you sure you just can't get over it?") can make things worse. We don't talk enough about how to handle these situations. For Naya, these interactions are also compounded by discrimination, making her desire to disclose that much more courageous. Even without adding the magnifying factor of having a known mental illness, about half of Black medical students report being watched more closely than their classmates, and about 66 percent said they needed to work twice as hard as others to get the same treatment and evaluation.[1]

I try to be better: "I'm so sorry that happened. It must have been hard for you to even share that information in the first place!"

"*Yes!* Well, my whole friend group talks about this stuff, and a lot of my friends are on meds, so I can share with them, which is comforting. But with other people or in a professional setting—it *is* hard. And when the premed advisors were giving me feedback at the end, they told me point blank not to disclose anything about my mental health—that I should keep it to myself unless it explicitly came up. I was a bit angry in the moment, but most of these advisors are deans or other powerful people, so I didn't react. Still, what they said is *super*-stigmatizing. Plus, to me, not mentioning my anxiety feels like lying. What do you think?"

"I get this question *a lot*," I tell her, maybe too passionately, thinking of my own recent therapy session during which I debated going public about taking Wellbutrin and maybe identifying with her a little too much. "My answer is: When it comes to telling these things, it's complicated." Like all things in mental health.

I based my unsatisfying answer on personal experience, of course, but research also suggests that revealing information about one's mental health can be risky. In one study,[2] directors of residency programs were asked to read mock descriptions of applicants, then evaluate each candidate. In one description, the "applicant" discusses having a history of depression. In another, the "applicant" writes about having diabetes. Diabetes and depression are similar in that they are both chronic conditions that can be managed with medications. The results showed that applicants who disclosed having a history of depression were less likely to get an interview compared to applicants who mentioned their diabetes, particularly if the former were "average" in other areas. In other words, disclosing about a mental health issue can affect the application process. And that's particularly true if a student is not among the strongest applicants to begin with, a category Naya might very well fall into given her MCAT score.

I remember when, all throughout my residency, I was reviewing applications for a spot in our psychiatry residency program. I assumed that of all the medical specialties, psychiatry would be the least likely to be biased against someone with a mental illness, especially because so many go into psychiatry as a result of family and personal experiences with mental illness. I was wrong.

I passed along applications to colleagues, and their reaction to seeing a self-disclosure was to groan and say things like, "Is it horrible that I wish they just kept it to themselves?" or "Not again." After those interactions, I even began to think that maybe psychiatrists are *worse* than doctors in other fields, because we understand more deeply what particular diagnoses mean. For example, we might applaud a medical student who had gone to an eating disorder clinic for treatment and, at the same time, know that being able to come out of treatment and be a resident the following year might be tough for that person to accomplish without relapsing.

When people are stressed, as so many residents are, they are likely to turn to their favorite coping mechanisms. This could make them backslide, and that outcome affects not just them but also the whole class. My colleagues voiced similar opinions about the student who was psychiatrically hospitalized in their recent past for depression or mania. I remember asking them if, by thinking that way, we were ourselves stigmatizing mental health, and someone said we were being *realistic*. I agreed, somewhat, but also pointed out that we are not their psychiatrists. If the applicant thinks they are ready (and presumably their treatment provider does as well), we should take that as fact.

I don't ever want my patients, Naya, or anyone else for that matter, to feel they can't tell their story, but if psychiatrists are potentially judging prospective residents with mental health issues, then what might the other specialties who have a worse mental health culture (like surgeons!) be doing?

No wonder so many healthcare professionals choose to remain silent about their own mental health issues. Granted, for people in medicine, there are fears of disclosing *any* disability. But the latest data suggest that more medical students *are* disclosing their physical disabilities so they can get necessary accommodations at school.[3] For illnesses like depression, however, the gap between the number of people who have it and those who actually disclose it remains as wide as ever.[4] This highlights a continued gap in seeking support for mental illnesses in particular, and yet another way mental illness and physical illness are not seen as the same.

———————

What I end up telling Naya in response to her question is slightly more nuanced. "There's some data to suggest that people can be biased against applicants with mental health issues, and I've heard examples from patients of people having their stories held against them or feeling like they were. But, I also strongly believe that if *you* want to talk about it, you shouldn't feel as if you can't. If someone holds it against you, do you even want to go to a place like that?"

I'm careful not to firmly tell her what to do either way, even if my inclination might be to advise her to say nothing, simply to protect her. Whatever her decision, I don't want her to hold the result against me or for me to unduly influence her.

"I honestly think my experience makes me more empathetic," Naya says now. "If you would've asked me, like four months ago, when all of this first happened, if I would ever appreciate any part of it, I'd have laughed in your face. But I realize that I've learned a lot about me and about suffering in general because of what I've gone through."

The data support Naya's belief. When individuals reflect on their struggles and experiences, that seems to improve measures of compassion and empathy.[5] Both are traits that I, for one, would want in a future doctor, even if their experiences led to lower test scores.

Naya sits up a little straighter. "I think all of this will make me a better doctor. Then again, I'm not even sure I'd want to go into a profession that didn't see it that way."

I agree with her, but I admit to myself that her response is a bit naive, as most jobs—regardless of the industry—are not exactly accommodating of mental health issues. This is despite the fact that depression is the leading cause of workplace disability worldwide.[6]

Still, there is a genuineness to her hope that I don't want to crush.

I proceed with caution, asking if she had, by any chance, spent much time shadowing other doctors. Naya laughs slightly and answers, "Yes, of course, and I know what you're hinting at. Lots of people seem burned out and unhappy, and no one is acknowledging it or even getting help. But that just seems ridiculous and bad for patients. Wouldn't it be better to just be open about what's going on, get help, and move on?"

I smile ruefully and say to Naya, "If only it were that simple. I think a lot of decisions medical professionals make are based on fear, or because of horror stories they've heard."

As much as I know Naya's version of the world is unlikely to materialize in medicine any time soon, I truly love this about younger people—the ones I teach and my patients. They're so idealistic, always cutting to the chase and wanting things to just be better, *today*. It can sometimes come off to the older establishment like they are complaining too much or don't get it, but they keep fighting anyway. It's beautiful, really. I was like that when I was younger, too.

They haven't yet learned that systemic and cultural changes don't happen overnight, if at all; they're willing to fight for something and believe they can make a difference. Unlike me and my contemporaries, they haven't waited for change to come, and then waited some more.

Feeling things so strongly, though, and then not seeing the change happen, can ultimately affect their mental health. It's one reason this age group has such high rates of mental health struggles. According to data from the Healthy Minds Network's survey in 2021–22,[7] more than 60 percent of college students meet the criteria for at least one mental health problem—a nearly 50 percent increase since 2013. Furthermore, 15 percent said they have seriously considered suicide, which was the highest rate in the survey's fifteen-year history. And while college is a hard time mentally for all groups, white college students are almost twice as likely to get help as Black college students.[8]

I see the reality of medicine peek through as Naya adds, "Is it true that when you apply for a medical license, the licensing boards can ask about your mental health history and if they don't like what they hear, you can be refused your license—or lose it?" she asks, and I immediately feel saddened that the lore has already spread to college students. "Is that one of the horror stories you're referring to?"

"Yes, though again, it's complicated."

The fear of losing one's license to practice medicine because of an admission of needing or asking for mental health help has significant consequences. According to one survey, 40 percent of physicians say they would be reluctant to get formal mental health treatment because of this fear.[9] In my visits with patients, and even in the question-and-answer portions of my national lectures, I spend a lot of time listening to healthcare workers' fears that stem from a horrible story they've heard, such as about someone having their license revoked or limited because of a mental health diagnosis or record of getting treatment. I can't help but think about what my friend whose physician husband died by suicide said to me, "Trying to get help doesn't usually result in getting help. People don't forget that you tried."

All these concerns about losing status occur despite the fact that the 1990 Americans with Disabilities Act says that, legally, potential employers can ask only about an applicant's current impairment due to a mental health condition. For example, it's okay to ask something like, "Do you currently have any condition that is not being appropriately treated and that could impair your ability to practice medicine with reasonable skill and safety in a competent, ethical, and professional manner?" What you can't ask is, "Have you ever been treated for or do you have a diagnosis of any mental health condition?"

Yet, many state licensing boards violate these rules, broadly asking about an applicant's past and current mental health treatment without taking impairment into account. This practice has lessened over time, however. In a study I coauthored in 2021,[10] we found that of the fifty-four states and territories in the United States, thirty-nine initial medical licensure application forms did follow the "only if impaired" guidelines and forty-one followed the "only current" impairment guideline. The numbers aren't terrible, but the fact remains that physicians who work in states that *do* violate these requirements are known to be more reluctant to seek help,[11] a reluctance that can persist throughout a doctor's career, which often involves moving from state to state. So far, in my own career, I've practiced in California and Missouri, and I had to obtain an Illinois license for telehealth to continue to see many of my current patients who live in Illinois and used to drive into Missouri to see me, but now can't. The Illinois insurance form (part of licensing) particularly sticks out in my memory; the question about mental health was nestled in with those about criminal behavior and pedophilia. As someone with a now public mental health history, I do often look at the wording and wonder, *Do I count?* And this problem is not exclusive to physicians; it's also an issue for nurses, social workers, and psychologists.[12] Healthcare workers shouldn't have to wonder what mental health questions are on a state's licensing form before they consider moving there for work. No one should be deciding between their career and asking for help, especially in a moment of acute need.

I decide not to go further on this subject with Naya, and I simply say, "I think you have to do what feels right to you. And, you absolutely should get help if you need it."

"I hear you. Oh, um, speaking of help, I probably should've written you. I know it hasn't been six months or whatever, but I haven't been taking the medication you gave me, Lexapro. I took it for about a month, but when it was time for a refill, I procrastinated, then realized that I didn't like how I felt on it anyway. Plus, I had this appointment already scheduled and figured I'd just tell you now. So I am."

"Okay," I say, not wanting to react in any way that might feel punitive. Side effects are absolutely a valid reason to change, or stop, a medication, and often the most common reason patients do so. "What were you feeling on it?"

"Weirdly, like I didn't have feelings at all."

"I've heard that from some people. Sometimes, I think it's because their feelings were so up and down before medication that *normal feelings* feel like no feelings. But it's also possible that, as you say, antidepressants can make some people feel a bit . . . for lack of a better word . . . blah."

"I just didn't like it. Sorry."

"No reason to apologize to me! Did you have any side effects coming off it? It can be gnarly stopping medication suddenly."

I know I've warned her about this, as I do all my patients; there is something called antidepressant discontinuation syndrome,[13] which happens in roughly 20 percent of patients. Symptoms can start within a few days, and may include feeling flu-ish, off balance, or experiencing insomnia, hyperarousal (anxiety, irritability, agitation), and nausea. The most common symptom I hear about, owing to how strange and frightening it can be, is something colloquially known as "brain zaps." People describe them as a feeling of electricity running through their head; they can last for weeks. That's why, ideally, antidepressants should be stopped with the help of a doctor.

Patients often worry that withdrawal symptoms are an indication that they have become addicted to antidepressants, but addiction is defined by long-lasting changes in the brain related to pleasure and decision making.[14] There is no evidence that antidepressants permanently alter the brain in this way. Instead, it's helpful to think about medication in a different way—the way a few patients have described it to me—as similar to eyeglasses. Like wearing glasses, on medications my patients explain the world looks different, and they just feel better and are able to function better in the world. But while they depend on them and prefer having them, that is not the same as addiction, whereby a person continues to use a drug at great personal cost and despite consequences to their health and relationships.

Naya pauses to think about her own experience stopping her

Lexapro, and then replies, "Oh, right, you mentioned that before—I felt okay, honestly."

"That's good. Are you wanting to try something else? Sometimes if one medication causes a side effect, another won't. A lot of this is trial and error, unfortunately. You still have many options to choose from."

"Can we not right now? I'm actually really good. I promise. I still have the propranolol and I use it occasionally, like before doing the mock interviews today, but I'm using it much, *much* less than before."

"That's a good sign, too. How often you need an as-needed indicates just how often you are feeling really badly. Does it help when you take it?"

"Yes, absolutely. But I have generally just been feeling better."

"That's great to hear, but just know that if your symptoms return, or you start using the propranolol more, medication is still an option, especially since I imagine you still have a lot of anxiety-inducing application-related events coming up. It's nice to just know there are some things we can do about that."

"It is." Naya replies.

"And a word of advice from one stressed test taker to another," I say with a smile. "Try to stay off social network conversations about applications and interviews. They tend to be full of people bragging about their successes, which can just make you feel bad about whatever is going on with you. I know it's hard to resist, but it's like self-esteem quicksand. Look for support and distractions, instead."

Once again, I'm speaking from experience. When I was applying to medical school, I worked at a nonprofit doing adolescent health policy with someone who also happened to be applying to medical school. Unlike me, she got into every school she applied to while I was wait-listed at many of the same schools. All medical schools do rolling admissions, which means that if someone turns down a spot, one opens up for someone on the wait list. I would often coyly ask if she was planning to go to all fifteen places or if she was going to start saying no to some, so people like me could get some good news. I swear I hated her for it so much. It felt as if she were collecting the whole deck of cards while I was hoping for a single card. As nice as she was as a co-worker, waiting while sitting next to her in that office was torture.

I want better for Naya than looking at what everyone else around her is doing and accomplishing, and feeling less than that in comparison. "I'll do my best to put up some boundaries," she promises. "I already told my roommate she can't talk to me about any of it," she emphasized.

"That's probably wise," I say, noticing that I feel proud of her—but also envious. I couldn't have done that at her age; it's hard to win if you don't compare.

19

"SO, HOW'S BEING back at work?" I ask hesitantly as Janet comes on the screen. She's sitting in scrubs and fidgeting with her mask, in what looks like a conference room. If I squint, I can make out the name of her hospital unit written on the dry erase board behind her.

"Fantastic, Dr. Gold, just FAN-TAS-TIC."

I play along with her sarcasm. "Oh, good, I'm glad it's been so easy for you."

She laughs slightly. "Ha! Yeah . . . in all honesty, so much has changed at work since I've been out on maternity leave that it couldn't possibly be easy. I think, on some level, I convinced myself that this—the pandemic—would all be over by the time I came back. But in some ways, it's even worse. Work is like a rude awakening, and I just keep thinking, *Oh, my God. This is our new normal.*"

"That seems to be a common, but hard realization for a lot of my patients recently," I tell her. It is November 2020, and as people have started to look ahead to the new year, many are struggling to adjust their definition of normal. "What does that all feel like to you?"

"I think it was a bit shocking at first, but now I'm just numb, like I have no emotions. Even when something should feel positive, and maybe has felt before, I just don't feel it anymore."

That happens to me sometimes, I think.

"Numbness can be an emotion," I tell her. "I'm not sure we think of it like that, but it's basically our brain protecting us from a flood of strong feelings so that, even if we can't physically run away from whatever is triggering us, we can at least escape psychologically." *Like me, when I numb out in an emotionally difficult session with a patient,* I think. I say to Janet: "We detach from our feelings, mostly unconsciously, to be able to deal with our environment and cope in the moment. It's something I see in a lot of healthcare workers right now because there's just so much to take in. It's a bit different from the compartmentalization that we learn to incorporate into our jobs to get by." Megan's face comes to mind for a split second. "This is more of a sudden emotional change in the face of something traumatic or right after; in your case, working in an ICU during COVID. It can sometimes feel easier to be numb than to let yourself feel all of it."

Even in the face of some of the hardest things we might ever witness or experience, we adapt. In fact, research suggests that the more triggers a person has, or the longer someone is exposed to a trigger, the less emotionally they respond.[1] We do what we have to do to survive.

Janet's eyes widen as she says, "I can recognize that something isn't right with me, and my husband can, too. But I also have a job to do. So, like I did during my first pregnancy, I figure, *I'll deal with it later.* I'll just take my antidepressant and not talk about the reasons *why* I feel like I do or, well, why I don't feel at all."

Many healthcare workers I see and talk to run on adrenaline, and they will keep running for as long as they can, so I'm not surprised to hear this from Janet, to whom I relay something Dr. Miller once told me: "The challenge with your method is that, unfortunately, you can only push your feelings down for so long, like a beach ball in water. They have a way of popping back up, with greater force, when you least expect them. Trauma does, too."

"I know exactly what you mean! The first week or so back on the unit, I was good and numb; I just put my head down and worked. I was even a little proud of myself for it. But then, just last week, I had to go into a patient's room to check on them. When I walked in, I realized I'd been in that room before I went on maternity leave. That was the same room where I did CPR on a patient, a pregnant woman, who later died. I was pregnant too, so obviously that stuck."

Now, the image was sticking with me, too. "Of course it would," I try to echo kindly. I can't help but reflect on the stories I have heard of doctors and nurses working with patients who are experiencing similar health conditions to them and they find it incredibly hard to continue to "just do their job," as Janet put it.

It's more than a matter of empathy for other people's suffering. I think about the psychiatric nurse with chronic suicidal thoughts, who struggled every time she asked patients—as she did every day— if they had them, too. And the doctor who was actively going through cancer treatment while taking care of a patient around her same age who had been hospitalized due to complications from cancer. Or, the nurse who spent all day working in an infertility clinic, where patients kept asking her if she had children of her own, not knowing that she was also struggling to conceive. These similarities make it hard for healthcare workers to put up boundaries and gain some emotional distance. No wonder Janet remembered the experience of her pregnant patient's death so viscerally.

Her voice quivers slightly as she continues. "I was in the room, and in my head I saw the pregnant woman lying there, dead in the bed, and her family outside screaming, even though they weren't actually there when it happened, because they weren't allowed to visit. Her face then sort of morphed into mine. When I finally came back into the present moment, I was gripping the door jamb, my knuckles were white, and I couldn't breathe. Luckily, the patient who *was* actually in the room was sleeping; otherwise what would she have thought? But my colleagues were around, and I *know* they saw me, especially when I stumbled out of the room and into an empty room, then strapped my arm immediately into a blood pressure cuff. I was scared that I was having some kind of attack—like something was really wrong with me. Reading my own vitals, I saw that my heart rate was elevated, but otherwise, medically, from what I could assess that quickly, I was apparently okay. It didn't *feel* like it, though. It was the worst feeling I've ever had."

"I can see how that would be scary. It sounds like a pretty realistic flashback with a panic attack attached."

"Yes. I think so, too. But it was so hard in the moment to tell real from imaginary. And even though I was scared and anxious, my predominant feeling was embarrassment. I mean, showing my crazy in front of people? And potentially in front of a patient? I don't do that."

I always find the words people use to describe their own experiences interesting. *Crazy* is one of those words that people with mental illness can find offensive and ableist, particularly when it refers to actual behaviors of someone with mental illness.[2] But at the same time, a lot of my patients use it about themselves, and I have to take their lead.

I probe for more from Janet, "Did your colleagues say anything?"

"Not exactly, but I guess I must've looked really bad, like a ghost, because people looked concerned, and someone brought me a glass of water. They were trying to be kind, but I don't like getting that kind of attention. I felt like they'd assume I was fragile or unfit. In a way, their caring made the whole thing worse."

"I know what you mean," I say softly.

"Did you think about telling them that?" I add, as I know from Dr. Miller that while there's no controlling what people think about us, if we can have a conversation about it, we can at least try to voice our side or put our worries to rest.

She looks down, embarrassed. "I just froze, I think."

"If it helps, you were just doing what biology tells all humans to do in a threat. Just like going numb, your reaction was a protective response to a threatening situation you couldn't escape or change. In the patient room, your body sensed danger and tried to get you out of it—the flight response. Which explains your heart rate."

Janet nods, "Yeah, like running the fastest fifty-yard dash I'd ever done."

I build on her metaphor: "Yes, but with a finish line that is constantly moving, as we have no clue when work will get back to normal. Or, worse, that maybe this *is* our new normal, where we are forced to be constantly running, seeing threats everywhere. But you can only do that for so long. It's why everyone is so exhausted, honestly."

Janet looks somewhat discouraged. "It feels kind of hopeless when you say it like that . . ." Suddenly, she looks as if she might cry, but she takes a deep breath and holds in her tears. I worry that I made everything worse in my honesty, but there is no way to sugarcoat a pandemic. "Like this won't get better and I won't get better, either. How can I, when healthcare is on fire, work is such a mess, and the stressors are just always there? It's pretty damn hopeless," she says.

Hope is critically important for a lot of reasons, but especially for someone like Janet, who has experienced significant trauma.[3] In contrast to *optimism*, which is defined as a general expectation that good things will happen, hope is about how we plan and act to achieve what we want.[4] It's the belief that it's possible to make things better, without distorting reality, and having hope not only promotes resiliency but also protects against mental health conditions.

In one workplace meta-analysis,[5] high-hope employees (defined by the validated measure, the Adult Hope Scale[6]) were 28 percent more likely to be successful on the job, and 44 percent more likely to report overall feelings of well-being. Measures of hope were also more predictive of academic achievement than factors such as intelligence, personality, or even prior achievement.[7]

Yet sometimes, especially in a crisis, hope needs to be cultivated. One exercise I sometimes suggest to patients like Janet is to think about all the things they are worried about and write them down. From that list, I ask them to figure out which ones they can actually do something about, focusing on what they can control, à la the serenity prayer. Those are the items I suggest they address, while letting the others lie. When things seem possible to manage, or even control, hope thrives.

The same goes for to-do lists. To help maintain hope, it's important not to fill your list with overwhelming tasks, like "write a book." It's best to stick with smaller, doable chunks like "write an outline" or "start chapter 1." Even getting to cross off "make a to-do list" counts toward hope. Instead of feeling unproductive and ineffective at the end of the week, as so many of my patients tell me they do, you at least get the smaller tasks done, even if the lists themselves are long. And completing tasks increases self-efficacy and, in turn, hope.

Before I can help Janet feel more hope, however, I do need to assess just how hopeless she is actually feeling. "It seems like a lot of things are contributing to your hopelessness," I say. "We can absolutely try to work on that together, but also, especially given your depression history, I need to ask: Have you been having any thoughts of ending your life?"

I ask because hopelessness is correlated with suicidal thoughts,[8] which is why it's an important symptom to notice and identify early. And contrary to popular belief, asking about suicide does not lead a person to more suicidal thoughts.[9] In fact, it may reduce rather than increase suicidal ideation and lead to treatment seeking. Patients often worry that if they talk about suicide to psychiatrists, they will be sent right to the hospital, which certainly isn't the case, at least not with me. Suicidal thoughts are actually quite common. What's most concerning is when the thoughts are new, or become more regular, or when people start planning how to do it.

"No, I could never do that to my kids or my husband. It never gets that bad. It never has been that bad, either."

"Okay, I had to ask. But please just pay attention to it, and maybe talk to your husband about doing that, too, and let me know if anything changes."

"Oh, absolutely. If I had those feelings it would scare me, so I'd definitely tell you, and him. One thing I will say, though, is that whatever I'm feeling has made it really hard for me to physically get myself to go to work and to stay there, too."

"What do you mean?"

"So, every Monday, after I get to work, I sit in my car in the parking lot, unable to get out. I just sit there with my heart rate increasing, crying for ten or fifteen minutes. I feel like my legs are heavy and I can't move, which means I'm late to every shift. I just don't want to go in and, after crying, I'm also afraid of having people see me like that."

"Is that the only place you feel like that? In the parking lot? Well, I guess that patient's room you mentioned . . ."

"No, I mean overall, I'm much jumpier, like someone dropped a clipboard yesterday and I actually yelped out loud. And I recently noticed that I'm triggered by the mask smell. I remember reading in a nursing textbook once that the way the brain is designed, there's a quick connection from the nose to the parts of the brain involved in memory, like the hippocampus.[10] That's exactly what happens to me. I smell the inside of the mask when I put it on, or while I am breathing in it, and immediately I feel like I can't breathe. Logically, I know that's not true, that masks don't cause trouble breathing, but I have that choked, breathless feeling. Like that patient had before she died . . ."

And now the picture is clear to me. "It sounds like you are now officially experiencing PTSD," I tell her, somewhat abruptly. I'd thought of that as a potential diagnosis during her last visit, but it was too soon to diagnose. I told myself I'd pay attention to see if it evolved. And it has.

"Sorry, what?" Janet seems to be having trouble following the conversation after telling me so many triggering stories, likely related to her PTSD and her drive to avoid triggers.

"I said I think you have PTSD."

Janet pauses and appears to be thinking about how that label sits with her. She says, "Can you have PTSD impostor syndrome? If so, I have that."

"What do you mean?"

"I mean no one has died in my family, and in fact I just added another member, so what right do I have to be so affected as just the nurse? So many people have it worse." Even questioning whether she "deserves" the diagnosis is emblematic of her having PTSD.

"I think there's always someone to compare yourself to, especially in your line of work, but that doesn't make your pain any less valid," I tell her. I've heard people call this concept the "grief Olympics," and I couldn't agree more. But we do ourselves a major disservice when we think our pain has to compare to someone else's. Competition makes no sense when everyone loses and is in pain.

Janet looks into my eyes; she definitely seems more focused now. "Deep down, I know you're right, but it's hard to admit it could be true, I think. I do know that I can't ignore what I'm experiencing anymore, and I need to do something—if not for me, then for my family. By the time I get home, I'm totally depleted—I'm just out of empathy. My older kid wants me to play, and instead I snap at her. It's not fair, plus I end up feeling so much guilt and negativity about myself, as a wife and as a mother." *More symptoms of PTSD* (from the category of changes in cognition or mood), I think to myself, affirming my diagnosis.

She takes a deep breath and continues, "And I just got back, and I'm already afraid I won't be able to stay. Sometimes, I wonder why I even bothered going to nursing school to begin with."

She's far from the only nurse that has said to this to me this week alone.

––––––––––––

As I'm writing this, the nursing field is experiencing a significant staffing crisis,[11] one that, like burnout and mental health challenges in healthcare, existed long before COVID and will continue long after. The new stressors created by the pandemic have only exacerbated the situation.

Take, for example, the rise of *traveler nurses*. Traveling nurses work in a temporary role, usually for short assignments, to fulfill staffing shortages in hospitals around the country. Because these nurses are hired to fill an urgent need, and the role doesn't come with the lifestyle stability that characterizes having a permanent job where you live, the pay tends to be substantially more than a typical hospital nursing job. Pre-pandemic, I had friends take those jobs just to travel and see the country, while working at different hospitals—something that, honestly, I was pretty envious of. Now, nurses are needed urgently pretty much everywhere, and traveling jobs offer something like a whole month's salary in a week—which makes them hard to turn down. They are definitely a hot-ticket item.

While nurses should absolutely be paid more, in general, this traveler's market makes it hard for hospitals to retain staff when nurses see people in similar jobs being paid significantly higher salaries. My nurse-patients have also told me that staff nurses are then often responsible for training and supporting the travelers, even if they are making substantially less. Although more hands are always appreciated for safe care, understandably this can lead some of my patients to feel undervalued by the system—another reason people leave (sometimes to take traveler's jobs), creating a vicious cycle. I always tell Dr. Miller that people can tolerate working really hard as long as they feel valued, but if they don't, it's nearly impossible to keep them. She tells me she told me that in the first place.

A thank-you is not enough. Or, even a gift during nurse's week. Particularly the ill-conceived gifts that I have seen from all over the country, like the piece of bubble wrap for stress reduction; an empty plastic bag that says, "I know this looks empty but it is filled with our love and support"; a lifesaver for "lifesavers" (we like a bad pun, clearly); or rocks. I wish I were kidding, but I could think of nothing worse to give a bunch of burned-out, frustrated nurses than rocks.

Inadequate staffing also leads to burnout, which is a prime reason nurses leave the profession. A large 2017 study[12] pre-COVID found that 31.5 percent of nurses who left their jobs cited burnout as the reason. So did an additional 43.4 percent of nurses who had considered leaving their positions. The pandemic only worsened this trend and increased the nursing shortage.[13]

Staffing problems also directly affect patients because patient outcomes are worse. For example, in one study of surgical patients, each additional patient per nurse was associated with a 7 percent increase in the likelihood of a patient dying within thirty days of admission.[14] In other words, it is not just about job dissatisfaction; it also includes patient safety and the quality of patient care. Nurses know that, which only worsens their burnout and moral injury.

Ultimately, when nursing suffers, healthcare also suffers. In fact, I have had ER physician-patients during these past few months tell me they were burned out not because of the pandemic but because of the nursing shortage. Another vicious cycle.

———

I hear the voices of my nurse friends and patients in everything Janet is saying. I find myself saddened that her time away from COVID, taking care of her newborn, didn't help her find her stride again, her love for what she does. But I'm also not surprised.

I want to tell her how important nurses like her are, and how needed. I can't help but think about the time when I was a resident on call and there were no beds in the call room. The nurses working on the psychiatric unit found me a cot and put it in an empty activity room for me to sleep on, without my asking for help. They didn't get to sleep on their night shift—that wasn't part of their deal—but they took care of me anyway, and always did (and do). They also always know what to do for patients, and perhaps most important, what not to do. It's no wonder nursing has consistently, for more than twenty years, been voted the most trusted profession.[15]

Still, my job isn't to be Janet's cheerleader, or even to tell her what to do. She's probably used to doctors and doctors-in-training trying to do that. And given that I'm a doctor, maybe she even has her own transference feelings toward me (a patient's feelings about a therapist or psychiatrist, owing to what they might represent in their life or past). This is different from countertransference, which is about the psychiatrist's and therapist's feelings triggered by the patient. I don't want to mess up our existing alliance, so instead I say, "It all sounds super-disruptive and pervasive in your life at this point. Even though there is something nice about fantasizing about leaving, I wonder: Can you hold off on making any big decisions right now?"

She pauses to think. "Yes, I think so."

"Our emotions can cloud these decisions, and any big changes might even make your symptoms worse, since times of transition can do that. Plus, trauma has no timeline. It comes out when you least expect it, and there's no clear linear pattern when it comes to healing from it. There are times you will feel better, and times you will feel worse . . . and this seems like a time you feel worse. So, if it's at all possible I'd love for you to not just rage-quit, or PTSD-quit, immediately. Of course, if you need time off for mental health leave, that's a different story . . ."

"Oh, I absolutely don't want that right now. I just can't. I'll keep it as an option, though, and appreciate the offer, honestly. It's good to have options."

"They give you hope," I say to her, but also me.

"I also think that starting some form of therapy with a clinician who has trauma expertise would be helpful. There are a few evidence-based therapies for trauma, like cognitive processing therapy (CPT), prolonged exposure (PE), and CBT (cognitive behavioral therapy) for trauma."[16] I tell her I'll send her a few links, which is one of the better things about being on my computer during the visit, and that she could always follow up via messaging.

She nods.

"And from my side of things, I think increasing your medication even more makes sense now, if you are up for it. It sounds like the increase from last visit didn't help enough, given all the symptoms you are experiencing right now. Luckily, the same antidepressant you take, Zoloft, can also help with PTSD symptoms. It's even FDA-approved for that use."[17]

"I think that makes sense to me. I want to get better, however possible, and I'm ready to take ownership of that. Another thing to check off the to-do list: Feel better."

We both smile.

I'm a big believer in medication, of course, but sometimes, for patients like Janet, who seem open to it based on the way they ask me questions or take feedback, I'll add some homework. I turn to this option especially with patients who don't have a regular therapist, as I'm acting in both roles for the interim. I make a choice to try that now, and slowly say, "In the meantime, until the higher dose of medication kicks in, I think you might find it helpful to do a self-inventory of sorts."

When I say this, I mean purposefully reflecting and checking in on herself—something we don't do enough. It goes beyond asking "How am I feeling?" or monitoring symptoms for changes, though that is essential and a good place to start. I explain the exercise and my rationale to her further: "It's clear to me that you spend so much time caring for others, at home and at work, that it's easy to lose yourself. The point of the exercise is to reflect on your values and look for ways to center yourself in them during the challenges of the workday or of parenting."

"How does that work exactly? I just think about what I value?" she asks somewhat skeptically.

"Sort of. I remember when I first started residency, they had us sort through a deck of value cards, and we picked out the ones that were the most important to us and also those that were the least. For me, the most were stuff like Family, Honesty, and Friendship, and the least like Power and Wealth. I remember looking around the room seeing what my co-residents picked, and wondering if they chose socially acceptable values preferentially, since we all could see them. One resident did pick Wealth as important, though, so maybe not." I laugh.

"Obviously, you haven't had time to reflect and don't have a long list in front of you, but does anything come to mind as important for you when I say 'values'?"

"Family, too, like you, but then maybe . . . Caring? Or Connection?"

"Those make sense based on what I know about you. If you go through the list, and I can send you a good link or you can just Google it, you can do the exercise fully yourself. It shouldn't take too long, but it's worth taking the time. Honestly, I still have the cards I picked as a resident, and they help ground me on even the worst workdays."

She continues to look like she is maybe just humoring me, so I add, "And, if you don't go the cards route, or that feels too formal or even too *out there* for you, you can also just ask yourself, 'What gets me out of bed in the morning?' Your answer is your mission, your *why*, and being aware of that matters. Even if you eventually still want to leave and find a different job, knowing these things will help you find a better fit."

Her mouth curves ever so slightly into the beginnings of a smile as she replies, "I hope." Which is, perhaps not coincidentally, also a value.

20

EVERY WEEK FOR the past month, I've gotten a B$_{12}$ shot and nonetheless, I feel the same level of utter exhaustion. And still, I keep hoping the next injection is going to be *the* one, the answer to my problems, the injection of energy that helps me get back to the way I was before. But even though my most recent labs suggest my numbers have gone up, in terms of my feelings and energy, nothing has changed.

Okay, that's an exaggeration. There has been one benefit: Being forced to leave my house once a week to go get my shot has been a boon to my pandemic social life. Except for my next-door neighbors, who are in my "bubble" and so invite me to dinner sometimes, seeing the staff in the lab to get my shot is pretty much all the in-person interacting I'm doing.

I start feeling frustrated, and before those feelings materialize, a song starts to creep into my head; it's one I turn to often in difficult moments, called "Fuck You," by Lily Allen. I consider it my theme song. I've turned to Lily Allen across all situations, from a stressful call shift to running a 5K courtesy of my med school mentor. "FUCK YOU, fuck you very very muuuuuuuch . . ." But even singing it at the top of my lungs now, or trying to dance it out (courtesy of Meredith and Christina, from *Grey's Anatomy*), doesn't seem to help. It's just another thing wasting my already depleted energy.

I've reached such a low point that even my house, once a haven, seems to be forcibly ejecting me. In these last months, I have had to replace my dishwasher; then my garbage disposal broke, upchucking chili all over my kitchen (it looked as disgusting as it sounds). Then I discovered that my mailbox was covered with ants—hundreds of them. Disgusted, I threw the mail on the ground and went looking for bug spray, then showered off my anxiety-induced itchiness. The next morning, when I grabbed my laptop, there were ants all over the floor, too. I turned to a nearby sprayer to solve the problem, and as I sprayed, my carpet turned white—I realized that I had accidentally spritzed bleach on my carpet. The spot is now a daily reminder of how my shit is absolutely NOT together.

In the weeks that followed, pipes above my living room ceiling developed a leak that left six inches of water, then I started finding dead mice: in my room, the garage, and even on the hood of my car. I was reminded of the Ten Plagues of Egypt from the Passover seder. The bad omens just kept piling up. I wanted to say to my house, "I don't want to be stuck here, either." But all I could muster was one word: "Enough."

I tell all these things to Dr. Miller, of course, and when she gives me a few seconds of silence—a pause that feels more like minutes—I am at least able to sit with it, a little less squirmy today. Finally, she asks, "So, how have you been feeling through all of this?" *Of course she did*, I think.

"Physically or mentally?"

"Both. They're both important."

"Well, I still *feel* horrible even though my B$_{12}$ is better. I'm just as tired, have a lot of trouble getting things done, and I'm constantly . . . *overwhelmed* is the best word for it. And my to-do list keeps growing."

"So, you're overwhelmed and having trouble with your to-do list?" she says, echoing what I just said, to reinforce my words and maybe also to check that she heard me correctly. At least that's what I'd do.

"Right. But it's beyond having trouble with my to-dos; I can't really do any of it. I'm realizing that if something doesn't need to

happen immediately, I put it out of my mind and focus on this minute. I swear I used to have more plans, and I remember regularly
thinking about the future and what I wanted to come next. I mean, I
was the girl who wrote my goals on the fridge! But now I feel lucky if
I can think beyond thirty minutes from now. I honestly have no motivation to look ahead, and even if I try, I feel overwhelmed by everything I have to do or should do. I'm getting really behind, and I'm
barely making deadlines with presentations and stuff, which is *so* not
me. I'm not sure if it's a great way of coping, either."

Dr. Miller looks me right in my eyes as if she understands my
experience completely. She says, "It's protective."

I can feel her caring for me as I sit on my couch. "What do you
mean?" I ask.

"Well, a lot of planning for everyone, including you, has failed, and
with things still changing every day, the future is really unknown. So, if
you only think about the present moment, it makes things easier."

As she says this, I think about how much I miss planning for the
future, and how I used to get mental health benefits from that—
from having something to look forward to. I'd even purposefully
plan things to do on the weekend or evenings if I knew I was going
to have a hard week at work. But not anymore. Things keep getting
canceled—like Taylor Swift's Loverfest concert or my friend's baby
shower. My attitude these days is: What's the point of trying to look
ahead? It's just another potential disappointment.

I ask, "This can happen unconsciously? The whole not looking
past the immediate present thing? Even if I used to actually like to
plan?"

"Sure, focusing on the now is the protective part. So, you avoid
the disappointment."

Our minds are weird, I think. I try all these coping skills on purpose, like journaling or mindfulness, but my brain does all these unconscious tricks of its own, too. I wonder if there are other things I'm
doing that I haven't noticed.

I sigh, then change the subject abruptly, getting to what's really on my mind. "I've been thinking. The B$_{12}$ shots aren't working, so obviously that was some kind of incidental finding. And, well, my doctor hinted that my exhaustion could be depression related, that I might be depressed, but I really don't think it's depression. I think I'd *know* depression." I realize I've said the word *depression* multiple times, in a kind of perseveration. "I mean, do you think that's what it is? Depression? Did I somehow miss it?" I notice myself speeding up as I go further down this line of questioning, with some mix of confusion and anger.

Dr. Miller confidently replies, "No, I think you're right that you aren't depressed. You've been depressed before, and as we've talked about a few times, this seems different. It *feels* different, even." The way she emphasizes *feels* I can almost feel it through the screen.

"I just don't get it. I know something is wrong with me, but I have no idea what, and no one else seems to know, either."

She pauses as if she's considering how to phrase her next words. Then she asks one pointed question: "You mean to tell me that you are a frontline worker, seeing frontline workers in a pandemic, and you don't know what's going on?"

I think long and hard, knowing that I must be missing something obvious. In my head, I start rattling off a differential diagnosis for fatigue (my iron, my sleep, my diet . . .) until it finally clicks, a click so loud it seems possible that it is audible outside of my skull.

"Oh, my God. I'm burned out!" I say, with the same surprise as the character Cher had in the movie *Clueless* when she realized she loved Josh. In other words, I'm floored, and I immediately start laughing. Like real, true, laughing.

Dr. Miller seems surprised by my response. She smiles and says, "What is the laughing about?"

I pause to take stock and try to understand my reaction before explaining. "I think it's embarrassing, and kind of ridiculous that I *literally* lecture on burnout regularly—in fact, I gave one yesterday. And people call me a burnout expert; and here I am burned out, and I had no freaking clue."

She smiles. "It's hard to see it ourselves sometimes."

Taking a step back, I know she's right, because the data agree. One of my favorite stats to bring up with my patients comes from a study of 1,150 surgeons.[1] Of those who had well-being scores in the bottom 30 percent of nationwide results, 70 percent believed their well-being was at or above average. In other words, surgeons (and other healthcare workers, I'm sure) who are truly struggling are likely to think they're doing okay or better than okay, because they can look around at their colleagues next to them at work and see someone who is sleeping less than they are or is as depressed as they are. They assume severe distress and symptoms like not eating, or not feeling joy about activities, are simply the norm in a stressful job like medicine. But just because burnout, insomnia, and depression are somehow the healthcare work-culture norm, that doesn't mean they are healthy, or right. It does make it harder to calibrate, though.

Beyond that, if these symptoms are a side effect of merely being in medicine, healthcare workers who admit to doing worse than others in terms of their mental health raise suspicions that they are somehow not cut out for the work. It's also hard not to wonder if something is wrong with you—if everyone else has the same stressors and symptoms, but they don't seem to have an issue powering through it.

All this is the culture of medicine, and it's partly why I didn't recognize my own suffering. Healthcare workers can go to all the lectures in the world on symptoms and diagnoses (or, in my case, *give* the lectures), but that doesn't mean they're good at applying to themselves what they learn or teach. Unless the signs become so obvious (and they are struggling so much), they're impossible to ignore.

With Dr. Miller's pronouncement, it's now hard not to rattle off the classic burnout symptoms in my head: workplace-associated emotional exhaustion, depersonalization, and decreased sense of personal accomplishment, and . . . say, *check, check, check. Guess I'm 100 percent burned out*, I think, still laughing a little, still embarrassed and very much incredulous. Of course, there were also the subtle signs, like changes in sleep and my schedule, or the anger at my inbox, that I blew right past and ignored.

Now that I know what's wrong with me and it has a name, I understand why some patients really like it when they finally have a diagnosis to go with their symptoms. It's validating to know that what you're feeling is real, that you aren't alone in it, and that maybe there *is* something specific you can do about it.

I ask Dr. Miller, "Is there a reason why I'm doing so much worse now? Nearly six months into this thing? It's not like something has suddenly changed." Just as I would with my patients, I want to understand the reason behind my burnout and the ever-important "Why now?"

"Have you ever heard of something called general adaptation syndrome?" Dr. Miller asks.

I shake my head. It sounded to me like something they teach in psychology training, but forget to teach us in medicine.

"I don't know if they are still teaching it, but from what I remember, when we experience high stress levels over and over, we think we're getting better at dealing with the stress, but we're actually habituating to it, physically, mentally, and emotionally."

"Uh-huh," I say, to prod her to keep going.

"But, at the same time, if we were suddenly thrown into that high level of stress, instead of increasing gradually, your body would be like 'Hell, no! This is too much! Make it stop!' It would be unbearable."

"Like a kind of stress exposure therapy?" I ask.

"Yes. Exactly! And it often looks like it does in you, with fatigue, burnout, sleep issues, poor concentration."

"I'm textbook." I smile and pose with my hands under my chin, as if my image was going into the textbook, too. She smiles back. More seriously, I ask, "But the whole time someone is dealing with that mounting stress, they have no idea? They think they're dealing with everything fine, until they're not, like it has been for me?"

"Yes, except unlike in exposure therapy, where the stress is limited—after all, you won't *always* be around a spider or an elevator, or spiders in elevators—because you're a mental health provider during a pandemic, there's no end in sight."

We both laugh, probably because we're both protecting ourselves from the actual underlying feelings of anxiety, or hopelessness, that could go with such a statement about our mutual predicament.

"This is like spiders in elevators on a plane—a phobia pileup," I crack, trying to keep the lightened mood going.

We laugh again.

But her assessment makes perfect sense. Suddenly, I'm no longer able to hold it all. So, I wonder, *Why am I so tired?* When, duh, of course I am tired, with the pandemic, work, loneliness, all of life right now. It just took a while for it to build up enough so that it was obvious. And then I go and forget a patient's name, and almost miss a talk, and fall asleep at 4 p.m., and it becomes impossible to ignore. I end my epiphany with Dr. Miller by saying, "I have to change something."

She nods. "There's a good quote by the author and doctor Rachel Remen that makes sense right now: 'The expectation that we can be immersed in suffering and loss daily and not be touched by it is as unrealistic as expecting to be able to walk through water without getting wet.'"[2] I happen to have saved this quote on my phone, after I noticed it on Instagram this week, so Dr. Miller's fortuitous words have special resonance. I wonder if she saw it on Instagram, too.

Dr. Miller knows I like thinking of quotes and poems to help me cope. In the past, she has texted me Mary Oliver poems, including one with an image of a bird over the words to "Invitation" on it. And I've sent her back some by poet and activist Cleo Wade, including a selection from a favorite poem called "How to Breathe When You Want to Give Up."

Sometimes other people's words do a better job of conveying how I'm feeling, just like sometimes someone else's eyes are needed to help diagnose what ails me. I continue, "I feel like this general adaptation thing is an analogy for the field of psychiatry. It's draining, like other medical specialties, but kind of subtly and untraditionally. It isn't the hours on your feet that drain you; it's the trauma in people's stories and the hate and the pain in the world that you hear about from dozens of patients over time. Over and over again."

"That makes perfect sense to me, based on my experience."

I sigh, and then I can't help smirking a little as I say, "So, I'm a burned-out burnout expert. Now what?"

"Now you have to try to do something about it."

21

I WOKE UP today thinking about *The Giving Tree*, by Shel Silverstein.

In the book, there's a boy and an apple tree. The boy plays with the tree, climbing on her trunk and eating her apples, which makes both of them happy. As the boy grows older, he spends less time with the tree, visiting her only when he needs things from her, like wood to build a house or apples to sell for money. Every time she helps the boy, the tree is happy. Even when she has nothing left but a stump for the boy, now an old man, to rest on, *she is happy*.

I grew up reading this story. In fact, I vividly remember referring to it in my bat mitzvah speech as an example of selflessness and giving. I didn't know it at the time, but in mentioning it, I was talking about some of my unhealthiest behaviors—ones I've carried with me to adulthood. Only recently, with the stresses of the pandemic, I've started to wonder: *Was the tree actually happy? And what would have happened if, just once, the tree had said no? Or, if it had responded Fuck this!?* Just like one of my favorite internet memes.

It may seem odd that the concept of helping others could be considered unhealthy, but in working with Dr. Miller, I now see that giving and giving and giving, and not leaving anything for yourself, will hurt you in the end. It's been hard for me to get here. Like most people, I usually feel good about dropping everything for a friend or working extra hours to help a patient who needs it. This behavior lines up with my values and my purpose in all my roles: as a sister, a daughter, a friend, and now a psychiatrist who is treating healthcare workers in the middle of a global pandemic. It's part of what makes me who I am and who I'm proud to be. It's what gets *me* out of bed in the morning.

But I've realized that, like the tree, I tend to help others at the exclusion of helping myself. There are times when even I can't deny that I'm tired, or sick, or emotionally drained and I need to listen to my own body and emotions and take a break. To put myself first. Or, at least, not last. Unfortunately, I still don't. I answer the direct message from a healthcare worker struggling and point them toward resources or I pick up the phone and help a friend's family member navigate a mental health crisis. Being the kind of friend I am has also led me to being in a few questionable friendships, including one where someone actually stole my prescription pad and got herself controlled substances. To the outside world, it might seem like I would do anything for someone I care about, but to quote Meat Loaf, "I won't do that."

Reflecting on these experiences, especially in the past few months, I've learned that helping others is as much a way to distract myself from my own feelings and struggles as it is an act of selflessness and meaning. Plus, since my work is inherently altruistic, and altruism is considered to be a good thing societally and culturally, I feel I have a stamp of approval to dive headfirst into overwork, subsuming my uncomfortable emotions and focusing instead on helping my patients and others. As a bonus, if I'm working all hours of the day, I never have the opportunity to stop and feel.

Something needs to change in my life. Because as I sit here, burned out, I'm as close to being a tree stump as it gets.

I hear so many of the same arguments from my healthcare patients. The expectation in medicine, particularly in a teaching hospital, is that you see patients, do research, teach medical students and residents, and do administrative work in between—and do all of it well. Many of these duties don't come with extra pay, including being "voluntold" to teach a class in your "free time," and yet somehow make up all the clinic hours you will have to miss. The demands often seem impossible to juggle, but then again, it seems like everyone else is managing. (If they're not, they're definitely not saying anything.) So, if I try to set some boundaries, saying I can't or I don't have time, it's easy to feel as if I'm somehow not doing enough. It's just me.

Beyond that, saying no to any request, no matter how busy I am, doesn't come easily for me. That's probably because it's diametrically opposed to my goals of achievement and perfection, highlighting my ever-present impostor syndrome. And so, I try extra hard, telling myself, "If I *can* do it, then I *should* do it." It doesn't matter if *can* means giving up my free time, or sleep. Saying no is for failures, obviously.

I also suffer from a severe case of FOMO—fear of missing out. I worry that if I say no, I might miss an amazing opportunity, in part because saying yes has sometimes led me to take new paths, like writing mental health guidelines for the media or writing an op-ed for a national newspaper with a brilliant co-writer I never would have met otherwise. The *yeses* pile up until there isn't an empty second left in my day. On some level, I must want it that way.

But it's completely unsustainable, and the pandemic has just brought everything to a tipping point—for me and for so many others. No matter how much I can achieve by saying yes to an opportunity, or how much FOMO it brings up if I say no, I'm learning that saying *no* is sometimes necessary, even if it feels uncomfortable. Sometimes I have to choose me, and it's not selfish.

Dr. Miller pointed out, and she was right of course, that I need to ask myself an additional question before I say yes to an additional demand: "Do I have the capacity to do it?"

It doesn't matter if the ask is prestigious or might help someone, if I don't have the emotional or physical bandwidth, I simply need to say no—or at least, no for now. I've even learned from a friend to make a "no list," jotting down every request I turn down. The point is to learn to feel as proud of those decisions as I am about the accomplishments on my CV. My no list is still small, but every paper I don't review or every talk I decline to give feels like a small win.

Like I've told Naya and so many of my college-aged patients, they will be better students if they take breaks, and I also believe that about me and my own work. But just as with so many things for me, *knowing* all of this is entirely different from actually doing it. Like so many of my patients, I had to learn this the hard way: By saying yes to something that I should've said no to, and then not doing a great job. Like the talk I showed up late for and almost forgot, or the last-minute writing of a popular-press piece that kept me up until 2 a.m. the night before the deadline, as I scrambled for expert quotes. Instead of blaming myself, I'm trying to learn from my mistakes and failures. To practice some self-compassion. Next time, I hope I'll be able to say no before dropping the ball. It's why Dr. Miller and I talk about this subject so frequently.

"I'm aware that work is called *work* for a reason; it isn't supposed to be fun," I tell her on one of our Thursdays. "But even some of the things I enjoy doing, like writing, are actually work. So, how do I turn it off and find the fun that has nothing to do with work?"

It's not that I haven't tried. I've turned off notifications, muted text threads, and blocked my email from updating automatically. I've even tried writing more realistic out-of-office replies, like: "I will probably see your message, because I have not yet figured out the perfect balance between how not to check my email at all, and how not to hate returning to an inbox number that results from that decision, which leaves me so overwhelmed it feels like I never went on vacation in the first place." While all that creates a barrier, giving me permission to say no, or at least a delayed yes, it doesn't fix the problem. I'm still missing something.

Dr. Miller replies to my question enigmatically. "Have I ever shown you the egg picture?"

"The what?" I ask, confused.

"The egg!" She's clearly excited. "Hold on; let me get a piece of paper."

I laugh and raise one eyebrow, a specialty of mine.

"Paper?! Have we entered a phase where you're going to draw for me? That's new!" Of course, many therapists have whiteboards to write on and illustrate a skill; I even had one in my office during residency for my CBT patients. But this is the first time Dr. Miller has ever used a visual illustration with me and, like her, I feel oddly excited by the novelty of it. Maybe because everything else in my life recently has felt like *Groundhog Day*. Sometimes, I worry that I'm boring her with the same old problems. I hope not.

"Ha! Well, I won't make it a habit," she promises, as she starts drawing a sunny-side-up egg with a yolk surrounded by a circle of egg whites. "Can you see this?" she asks, holding the paper up to the screen.

I lean in and nod.

"So, the yolk, that's work—meaning all the work you do, the patients, the advocacy, the writing, all of it. It goes here, in the center," she says, pointing. "The white part is bigger, and that's everything else—your close relationships, your family, your hobbies, your fun."

"Okay," I nod.

"But for you, the yolk is just oozing all over everything."

I smirk a little. "Like when you cut into eggs Benedict?" I like the analogy because I like my food, but it also makes perfect sense to me: My egg whites, which supposedly are the healthiest part, are struggling to stay pristine.

"Exactly! So, the idea is to figure out how to spend more time in the white part by figuring out more stuff you like."

"To balance it out. And, I guess, to balance me out. If only I knew what to put into the white."

"Well, anything you want to do that you enjoy—I can't tell you exactly what those things are." *Oh, how I wish she could, or even would*, I think.

She then asks, as she often does before we go, what I'm doing for myself that week. It's a question I need to be asking and answering.

"I think I'm just trying to figure it out by doing things I used to like doing but haven't done in a while. Like reading a book for fun, or drawing." I start to think, then, about how I love art and miss it. When I was younger, art was my favorite class and I would copy Disney cartoons pretty decently. My house is also covered in cool paintings I've bought from street artists whenever I travel, like the street scene from Paris or a pineapple drawing from Cuba. I even have what basically counts as a whole gallery of works done by a professional artist who happens to be one of my best friends from elementary school. As kids, we would draw together in her garage. I say to Dr. Miller, "I'm just trying to find the fun in all of that again. To make me more than work."

"You've always been more than work. You know that, don't you?" she tells me, gently. "It's just easy to forget that, especially now."

22

"I'm HAVING A lot of realizations lately. I blame you," Megan says with a wry smile, as she pushes back her headband over her silver-gray hair. It's been around a month or so since I've seen her last.

I smile. "What do you mean by that?"

"Well, a few weeks ago, I had a medical student who saw her first code in the ER, a kid actually, and she started crying right after. I said to her quietly, 'Come outside with me to get some air.' She looked back at me skeptically, maybe because I have a resting bitch face. But truly, I was trying to give her space to feel whatever she wanted to feel, including the freedom to cry if that's what she needed. In other words, to do what no one did for me."

I think back to the story she told me of her own first code experience, and immediately feel empathy for her and this student. So many things in medicine are inherently emotional, and yet doctors mostly aren't given the time or space to acknowledge them. We get desensitized, and maybe even dehumanized.

Codes are a good example—one I think of as a missed opportunity. Even if hospitals have structured debriefs for students and staff after someone dies, these rarely focus on anything other than what was done technically and what could have been done differently. While those debriefs can reduce stress and improve patient outcomes,[1] the focus is generally not on the team's feelings about the experience. Some institutions, however, are doing better, incorporating what is known as a *pause* after a patient dies. It lasts only a minute or so, which is about the shortest time I've ever heard of for processing, but it's meant to allow clinicians an opportunity for reflection before moving to the next task. As brief as it is, studies show that it can be an effective tool for honoring the moment and allowing some closure. A grief ritual, even. It also has been shown to increase doctors' professional satisfaction and decrease their distress.[2] Honoring the pause as a group also helps clinicians and staff feel less isolated in their experiences and emotions. I've been told by patients of mine who work in the emergency room that these moments of silence have really saved them mentally. It would be great if this were done everywhere, for every code (not just deaths!), but we aren't there yet. Still, it's amazing to think that such a tiny ritual could create such an impact, and even change the culture of medicine. Bright spots like this give me energy to keep doing the work I do.

Megan continues with her story. "The thing is, no matter what I said, this medical student kept trying to hide the fact that she was crying. She'd wipe her tears, duck her face, all of it. Even after I said, 'You just saw someone die; give yourself space. It's sad. It's not normal that none of us are crying. It just isn't.' I was completely sincere, speaking from the heart, and trying to normalize the experience for her, but instead of hearing me, she kept on saying, 'It's just allergies. My allergies are bad. I'm totally fine.'

"I knew this was not true, so I said, 'Listen, take a breath, it's okay. You don't have to tell me anything and you don't need to explain. I just want you to have a moment to breathe and not feel ashamed.'

"And she still said, 'It's fine. It's my allergies.'"

"It sounds like you were really trying to help, and honestly it shows a lot of growth on your part in the language you used, and even that you tried to do it at all. It seems like maybe she was embarrassed and didn't know what to do or say. Maybe it wasn't about you, and more about the culture of medicine in general. How did you feel afterward?"

"On the one hand, I understood that she could have thought I was singling her out, instead of trying to help. Maybe she even thought it would affect her grade. On the other, I felt like I failed. It honestly made me want to give up and go back to my resting bitch face. At least I wouldn't be invested then."

"It's *so* hard to change the system when you're viewed as being a part of it," I told her, sympathetically.

"Oh, yeah, absolutely, but maybe, ironically, the system was never built for people like us in the first place. The culture of medicine is very masculine, and how doctors are supposed to show emotion is rooted in that. The gold standard is to be able to work through any-thing and everything. I mean, the founding fathers of medicine worked so hard and so often that they were all addicted to drugs to stay awake and do the work with the hours required by the end of it. It's sad if you think about it. That's what our culture was built on. I was just trying to give the student some of the hardest commodities to find in our field: time and space."

"And support, which matters even more than you might think."

Despite Megan's experience, supervisor support is one of the most significant protective factors against healthcare worker burnout. In a large study of more than 57,000 health system employees,[3] the higher a supervisor's composite score for items like making people feel empowered on the job, treating people with respect and dignity, and recognizing people for a job well done, the greater the chances employees felt satisfied—and the less likely they were to experience burnout. Data since the pandemic have shown a similar correlation: In one study at a large New York hospital system, higher perceived support from hospital leadership translated to a lower risk of PTSD, depression, and general anxiety disorder in healthcare workers.[4]

The question I always get is, "What exactly is a supportive supervisor?" While there is no clear-cut definition, it's a good sign if employees *feel* supported, subjectively, and feel able to ask for help.

Unfortunately, most supervisors are not taught about the best ways to communicate with their employees about mental health and emotional needs. One study by Deloitte[5] found that just 22 percent of line managers had received some training on mental health at work, even though 49 percent thought it would be useful. So, like Megan, most end up feeling unprepared to do the job, and 86 percent noted that they would think twice before offering help to a colleague whose mental health concerned them. This trickles down to employees, and as a result, more than a third of employees did not approach anyone the last time they experienced poor mental health.

Having had the privilege of seeing teachers and their students, supervisors as well as their employees, in my clinic as patients, I have the unique chance to hear perspectives from all sides of a situation. I see the person who feels unheard or judged by a supervisor who reacted in a particular way to their mental health needs, and I hear from the supervisor who feels like they did the best they could and yet could tell they hurt the employee. From wherever they are standing, the fact that healthcare doesn't teach us how to deal with emotions in the workplace affects all parties significantly, increasing rates of burnout, as one person passes it on to the next, like a contagion; data has shown this to be true in workplaces with high rates of emotional exhaustion, like healthcare.[6] That makes sense, though, as a burned-out supervisor might take it out on their employees, being quick to anger or, at the very least, less supportive than they might otherwise be. In these past few months, many trainees have told me that their attendings no longer had time to mentor them or answer questions, and were more irritable or frustrated when asked. They tell me these doctors seem as if they are barely getting through the day, which is scary for them to see. To make it past the toughest training years in medicine, it's imperative for residents to tell themselves that things will get better, but resident-patients of mine tell me that they're now starting to doubt that happier future, and as a result, to doubt their future in the field at all. That doesn't bode well for the future of the workforce, or the health of it.

Megan is starting to fight against that. She tells me, "I guess I just wanted to show this student that you can be a doctor and let your human side show. I believe that now, working with you, and now also my new therapist. Both of you have made that clear to me."

"How did we do that?" I ask, not for the praise but to have her put words to her own growth.

"I think you gave me permission to feel, and helped me realize that my feelings count, too, and not just a patient's feelings. All that has helped me feel less negative about myself—the negative feelings we discussed last time—and less numb."

"Oh, that's great. I'm so glad your therapist and I are on the same page. And that you found one. But also remember, they aren't *negative* feelings—they are just *feelings*." I notice I'm sounding a bit like Dr. Miller as I say this. Suddenly, a quote from Mr. Rogers pops into my head, one I regularly use in lectures to healthcare workers. I decide to relay it to Megan: "There is no should or should not when it comes to having feelings. They're part of who we are, and their origins are beyond our control. When we believe that we may find it easier to make constructive choices about what to do with those feelings."

We pause, considering that, and I ask another question reminiscent of Dr. Miller: "Have you been able to practice pausing and naming your feelings?"

"A bit, yes, though it's easy to forget if I'm overwhelmed by work. I'm trying to prioritize it because it doesn't take long. I'm also using the *feelings wheel* my therapist gave me to broaden my vocabulary." I immediately picture a circle divided up into pie slices with ever more descriptive words for general emotions. For instance, in the "sad" slice, there's also *lonely, depressed, shameful,* and *isolated.* This is a tool I often use with patients who have trouble finding the words for their emotions, which is common in healthcare workers who may have become *alexithymic,* a fancy psychiatric term meaning they can't actually identify or describe emotions in themselves (or others, for that matter). Maybe that's because most doctors are never encouraged to feel out loud in the first place. Megan elaborates. "Now, if I feel angry, I sit with it and think more about what kind of anger it is. Like, am I frustrated or furious?"

I smile, unable to mask my pride in seeing such concrete changes in her. "And does that help?"

"Yes! I'm not just *okay* or *fine* all the time, but I'm also not an angry person and I'm not a sad person. I'm just a person who is reacting to situations with a particular emotion. There's nothing bad about that. It just is."

I empathize, and continue to be impressed. "It can be a hard thing to not try to suppress or change a feeling, can't it? For me, sometimes the answer is to not do anything. Just be angry if you are angry. Let it out. Try not to turn right to a coping skill to make it stop, but stay with it."

Anger, like sadness, has a purpose. Like in the animated movie *Inside Out*, which I tell Megan is a must-see, because it describes experiencing emotions so well, including the importance of "negative" ones like sadness or anger. I recommend it often.

"Thanks for sharing. It helps to know that you're dealing with this stuff, too, and to hear some actual tangible things that have worked." In that moment, I realize I am doing for Megan what Dr. Miller does for me by self-disclosing: helping her feel less alone.

Megan adds, "I did mention earlier that I'd had some *realizations* plural. The other one is that I cried in front of a patient. You would be proud of me, I think."

"What? That seems huge! Tell me more about it."

"Well, I was finishing with someone in the ER, and as I was leaving the room, I noticed this teeny woman staring right at me. She was maybe seventy years old, and she came up to here on me," Megan says, gesturing to the middle of her chest.

"I didn't recognize her, so I walked over to see another patient, but she came right over and stood right in front of me, staring. I said, 'Can I help you?' a little irritated. She replied, 'You're the one who cried and held my hand when my husband died.'"

I interject, without even realizing I'm stopping the story. "Wait, she saw you cry?"

"Yes! I had trouble placing her, but then I remembered the day her husband died, about four years ago now—it was suddenly as clear as if it had happened yesterday. It was just a horrible day altogether, and his death was the last straw. He reminded me a lot of my dad, who was also sick at the time."

"You don't have to justify it. You surprised me, that's all." In our first session, Megan had told me she hadn't cried in years. Maybe it was a smaller amount of time than she remembered, or maybe she just didn't notice, as she had become so disconnected from her emotions. "Not to belabor the point, but how did you feel when she pointed that out in the middle of your workplace?"

I hoped, in asking about her feelings again, she wouldn't become irritated with me for persisting on the topic, as I know I sometimes do when Dr. Miller does this, especially if I just want to talk about something else entirely.

"I felt, and probably looked, embarrassed and uncomfortable. Those are the words that come to mind. At first, I wanted to deny it. *Crying? No! Absolutely not. You have the wrong person. You want the other tall gray-haired woman ER doc.* But I also didn't want to lie and send her searching for someone who didn't exist. So instead I just started walking to my patient's room again, hoping to cut the conversation short with *really important doctor stuff.*"

"Ah, yes, the best excuse that no one dares to challenge—a patient *needs* me," I nod, commiserating. I've used that ploy myself when there are phone calls and texts I don't want to continue.

"She didn't let me get away, though. Instead, she reached for my hand and said, 'I want you to know that you doing that was the most important interaction with a doctor I had that day. Maybe even ever.'"

Megan takes a deep, shaky breath. "When I heard that, I . . . I just lost it. I started to cry right then and there, and tried to hide my face with my hair, but she actually reached in and pushed it aside so she could see me. It felt comforting, somehow. Then I told her, 'You don't know how much that means to me. I always try to hide the fact that things at work affect me.' And, she said, 'No, no, patients need to know that doctors have a heart.'"

"Wow," I breathe.

"Right? I wanted to tell her that my psychiatrist would agree with her, but . . ." she smiles, "one revelation at a time."

After a pause, she continues. "At that moment I decided I never want to feel bad for crying again. It's like this woman gave me permission to be the *real* me." I'm reminded of another quote, this time attributed to one of my favorite authors, Charlotte Brontë: "Crying does not indicate that you are weak. Since birth, it has always been a sign that you are alive." This one I keep to myself, despite its power. One author quote is probably enough for any session.

"So now you're okay being a doctor who cries?" I ask, reflecting back what she has just said with encouragement and not judgment. I'm acutely aware that this is important for her and is a signal that the numbness and difficulty feeling emotions that brought her to see me in the first place have improved, at least in part because of our conversations. I also wonder if I feel the same—that it's okay to be a psychiatrist who cries in front of colleagues or patients—and honestly don't know the answer. I wish I did.

Megan answers passionately, "That patient showed me that what I'd always thought was inappropriate was actually the exact right way to help her. To be the doctor she needed."

I jump in, "Our patients are often the best teachers. If it helps, I think most of the patients I've talked to, especially the ones who end up seeing me after a bad experience with a doctor, prefer their doctors to be real. To understand and empathize with them. To feel out loud even."

The data agree with what I've seen in my office. Physicians regarded as more empathetic earn higher patient satisfaction ratings.[7] They also have better diagnostic and clinical outcomes[8] and are less likely to be sued than doctors who don't seem empathetic.[9] As an empath myself, data like these make me feel good, especially on days when my bones hurt from absorbing the pain of other people's stories. That's when I try to remind myself that it really helps people that I am the way I am, even if I haven't cried in the office with them yet.

"It did feel affirming," Megan nods. "Honestly, it's so rare that I'm thanked or complimented by patients. There's something really nice about it."

I find myself drifting to something Dr. Miller said when I got her a present for the holidays—a signed copy of a book by the poet Maggie Smith, *Keep Moving: Notes on Loss, Creativity and Change*. As we over-analyzed the gift giving, just like I knew we would, she asked me if I did it because I wished people thanked and appreciated me more. Now that I think about it, the answer is probably yes.

There is something nice about being appreciated by patients, but when it happens, I'm all too likely to smile and forget about it. Like many people, I have a tendency to let negative events affect me more strongly than positive ones. This is called *negativity bias*, and it's no accident. Evolutionarily speaking, noticing the bad, dangerous things (for example, poisonous berries or incoming predators) increases our chances of survival, so it makes sense that humans have inherited genes predisposing us to pay attention to and remember potentially harmful things in our environment.[10] And if we happen to be stressed or overwhelmed, we're apt to zero in on the negative even more. Except what was once adaptive is now likely to perpetuate a downward spiral of exhaustion, anxiety, and depression, especially in people already struggling with those things. It's too easy to zero in on one snarky comment on social media, or the one question you missed on an exam as if the rest don't exist.

To Megan, I say, "It's important to see the good in what we do—helping people, supporting them, getting a diagnosis right, whatever it is that works. It helps us survive even the worst of things."

"Oh, my gosh—yes," she says, nodding vigorously. "In residency, I was so buried in the negative that I couldn't see the good anymore, and it took a huge toll."

Finding the good, seeing the meaning in the work we do, is crucial to preventing burnout.[11] Holocaust survivor and psychiatrist Viktor Frankl described human beings' primary motivation as seeking meaning and purpose, not pleasure or power. In his book *Man's Search for Meaning*, he wrote, "Those who have a why to live can bear with almost any how." In a lot of ways, he was right. In a survey of 2,000 family physicians, feeling a sense of career purpose is the factor most strongly associated with happiness;[12] it's also associated with decreased mortality.[13]

That's why I sometimes try to tell patients, like Megan and Janet, to reflect on what gives them meaning in their day, or to at least think of the things that give them energy rather than deplete them. Studies show that physicians who spend less than 20 percent of their time engaged in meaningful activities—say, doing insurance paperwork or writing notes in the electronic medical record, as opposed to seeing patients or mentoring—report higher rates of burnout.[14]

Compared with doctors in other specialties, I have a more flexible schedule, so I try to arrange my time so that the meaningful stuff balances out the less satisfying work. This could mean being sure to not schedule all my horrible meetings on Mondays or giving myself some flex time to decompress after what I know will be a difficult session. That's harder for doctors in training to do, or for someone in emergency medicine, like Megan. Still, making a point of recognizing some of the good in what we do is at least a start.

This is why I tell her, "You might want to think about actually pausing at the end of your day to reflect on the good things that have happened. You can journal about them, or record them on your phone, or even use a text-messaging program from Duke University that will give you prompts."

Megan looks skeptical, but I have receipts. According to studies on healthcare workers, those who participate in the texting program for fifteen days straight report improvements in emotional exhaustion and depression and feel more happiness even up to a year later. Especially the people who felt the worst at the beginning.[15]

"But isn't that like saying, 'Let's forget all of the bad and pretend there's only good?' You know—toxic positivity?"

Her question activates an almost automatic response in me, because I get it from patients so often. "I think it's different. Consciously reflecting on the positive can help us balance our preoccupation with the negative, because we are then able to recognize the good along with the bad. It's not just thinking about the positive and only the positive, or somehow refusing to see the bad. Just because you focus on the forest and not the trees that doesn't mean you forget that the trees exist."

What I'm trying to tell Megan is that nothing is all good or all bad. There is often a middle ground between the two opposites. In the field of psychiatry, we like to use the word *dialectics* to describe this way of thinking: the ability to view something from multiple angles. There is an entire type of therapy, called dialectical behavioral therapy (DBT), that is built on this principle. In Megan's (and my) case, it would involve normalizing and validating how difficult medicine is, especially now, while also reflecting on the good things about it. Another thing I need to work on myself, I guess.

Megan sounds only slightly more convinced when she says, "I guess I just really hate the idea of 'Don't worry, be happy,' or good vibes only." I can tell she is trying not to be overtly sarcastic or dismissive.

"Oh, me, too. In the extreme, that kind of positivity can feel really ridiculous, especially when you're struggling. My therapist once said to me that the goal in life, and of therapy even, is never to just be happy. Actually, she said something like, 'Happiness isn't the goal, because happiness all the time is unattainable and unrealistic.' That struck a chord with me."

"That's *so* true. But those stupid hats and shirts people wear with those slogans on it suggest otherwise."

I personally prefer the honest slogans, like my hoodie that says, "It's OK not to be OK all of the time." I try to show my own skepticism through humor, and I say to Megan, "I guess they could say something like 'Don't worry, be neutral,' or 'Good and bad vibes—both are welcome,' but I'm not sure how good that would be for business." We both laugh.

"If it helps, at the end of the day, you can also write down one crappy thing and three happy things, so you can still get some venting in . . ."

"Okay. You win. On Monday, I'll try the crappy and happy version, and if I like it maybe I'll try it with the team, too. Eventually, if they handle it and like it, maybe we'll even skip the crappy. Baby steps."

"Look at you becoming a champion of well-being."

"Well, *someone* has to be," she smiles.

I smile, and promise, "Just starting to have these conversations will change the culture tremendously. People will start to see you as a person to go to for support." As I say this, I think, *Like they do to me, though maybe it's more expected in psychiatry.* "And, if you only end up doing it for yourself and not your team, that's just as important. How *you* are doing matters, even if it's not as tangible as introducing the exercise with others. Because you are still changing the culture. Getting help is good leadership."

Suddenly, an idea pops into my head. "I don't know what you'll think of this idea, but I keep a box of the things patients have written or given me—I'll scribble down something nice they've said on a piece of paper, and stuff it in the box."

I think about my box, buried in my home office on the back of a shelf, and what's in it. There's a picture of my old dog that a patient drew for me. I was seeing her in the hospital and she was at the height of a manic episode, showing symptoms of "increased goal-directed activity." She had drawn a bunch of dogs that visited the unit as emotional support animals, and I complimented her on them, so she asked if I had a pet she could draw. I thought about just printing any pet to give her more photos, because . . . boundaries, but something stopped me. I said yes, and I printed her a photo of Leo, my Maltese/Yorkie mix. After he died, my looking at that drawing made a difference.

There's also a letter from the parents of a patient, thanking me for helping her improve so much that she was able to safely go back to college. And one from a long-term therapy patient I saw at the end of my training, thanking me for helping him feel comfortable talking about his emotions. Then, there are letters from a whole class of residents I taught when I was chief resident. Each wrote me a different letter and labeled them for different uses, like the one that says, "Open on the first day you teach," or "Open on a Bad Day." Somehow, this group intuited the right kind of gift for me.

Megan seems intrigued, so I go on. "When I'm having a bad day, or I start to doubt why I do this, or I wonder if I'm even good at it, I look through it all. I call it 'my box of positive reinforcement.' But it's really about finding meaning. I have healthcare-worker patients who do it, too, but have spread the positive reminders throughout their office, in books randomly, or in drawers. So, it's a surprise when they find something—but the good kind of surprise."

"Sounds like I could use that most days."

I think about how I agree, and that I should probably go through my box again, as I could use a pick-me-up. It's so easy for me to get laser-focused on the patients who aren't improving (or the time I forgot someone's name!), or the ones who are pissed off if we have to cancel a session for a rare sick day ("I know you have an emergency, but . . ."). It's too easy to forget the good we can do.

That is, until we have a patient like Megan, who is not only improving herself but is also trying to help her team and her patients. It's hard to not find purpose in helping people who help people. They pay it forward, and in a sense through my work, even if sometimes I feel like a tree stump, I'm actually exponentially growing branches. Each one is another person I've helped, even if I've never met them.

Healing the healers affects us all. I'm working on remembering that.

Conclusion

THIS PAST WEEK, I was asked to give a talk on burnout to some heads of a medical division in the hospital system. The two women physician leaders told me they wanted me to use an amalgam of my previous talks and slides, kind of like an audition, before speaking to their group of employees. Even though I've given these talks dozens of times, I prepared for the meeting, then went through my presentation as the two women listened politely, along with their administrator, who had invited me in the first place.

The talk took about thirty minutes, and after I was done, I paused, expecting to get some feedback. The room was silent—like, really uncomfortably silent. They told me they'd be in touch.

A few days later, I got an email from the administrator asking me to call him, which didn't feel like a good sign. When I did, he told me that they had been considering having me speak to their department, but that it wasn't going to work out after all. Clearly, something was off, and after some coaxing on my part, he told me the truth: "They didn't think you were serious enough to give the lecture."

Before my head could absorb his words, or my negative self-talk could get in the way, I burst out laughing.

He tells me he is surprised that I'm "so unfazed."

"To be honest," I say, "if someone had said this to me in medical school, I would have cried and tried to change myself. I would have thought I'd failed and was a major disappointment. But now, I know my authenticity is my superpower."

In some respects, my response hearkened back to when I was just starting out on my path to medicine. Back then, I prided myself on not fitting the mold because of my lack of a filter, my preference for humor and sarcasm, and my ability to recite the names of the entire cast of *Jersey Shore* more confidently than I could name most types of infectious diseases. There were so many times as an undergrad, in medical school, during residency, and even now, as a fully formed attending, that I looked around and felt like I was a teenager and everyone else was a grown-up, and that if I was going to be successful, I'd better try to mold myself into something I wasn't (a bona fide doctor).

No wonder I hated being both premed and a medical student, and I constantly thought about dropping out or doing something different. I know now that fantasizing about *any* other job is a subtle sign of burnout, but at the time I just felt a cloud of doubt above my life.

I never acted on that doubt, or let it persuade me to try something different, because the negative self-talk in my head also kept telling me that if I quit medicine, I'd be a failure. I think all medical professionals probably should question their decision to enter healthcare multiple times along the way, because of the time and energy investment, and the fact that so many don't probably accounts for some of the high rates of distress in this group. I just started a little late and wondered a little less seriously. Obviously, I did stick with a medical career, even though I often didn't know why, or even if it was my choice to keep going at all. I regularly questioned, and still do, if I was staying simply to please others or live up to everyone else's expectations.

And somehow, in spite of my best efforts to remain the nonconformist, joke-cracking person I'd been proud of, I let medicine change me. I had to, or I wouldn't have survived the broken system.

But when I laughed at the rejection from the administrator, I caught a glimpse of who I was before, and I liked it.

A Taylor Swift lyric started to repeat in my head, "I'd like to be my old self again, but I'm still trying to find it." I have never related to a lyric so much.

I am, after all, trying.

———————

Recently, I was being interviewed for an article on the mental health of healthcare workers. I'd said yes to this request because I want people to hear the stories of my patients, to know what they are experiencing now and what they are likely to experience in the future. I feel honored to be able to do that, and I find a lot of meaning in advocating for people like Luke or Janet.

The reporter asked me, an expert on burnout, for its definition, signs, and symptoms. He also asked what people can do about it and how the healthcare workplace presently is contributing to the problem. The answers were easy for me, as I teach about them and think about them daily.

Then, as the interview was winding up, the reporter suddenly asked, "Out of curiosity, and you don't need to tell me if you don't want to, but how has this experience been for you?"

His question took me by surprise. In truth, I choked a little on my water. I felt my face flush, and I noticed that I felt confused, and maybe even a little violated. Like the expert third wall had been broken and instead he had classified me as another healthcare worker suffering through a pandemic.

Do I want to tell him my truth? I wondered. I knew I didn't owe it to him or to anyone else to talk publicly about my experiences. I'd simply be protecting my privacy, which is different from worrying about stigma. On the flip side, I worried that if I didn't answer, I was being inauthentic. That same worry I'd discussed so many times with Dr. Miller. In my mind, that went against everything I was learning and working on.

Maybe this is how change happens, I remember thinking, and before I could filter myself or think about what was an appropriate level of vulnerability, I poured out my story, confessing everything I'd struggled with over the last six months. To a complete stranger. With a recording device.

I could no longer keep it a secret. I could no longer give in to the shame. "Well, I'm a burnout expert, and I'm slowly recovering from burnout."

He tried to remain expressionless over Zoom, but his face showed a mix of surprise and intrigue. If you'd asked me how I was feeling during that conversation, I'd have said *empty* or *emotionless*. Just a storyteller conveying the details of a story, yet so disconnected from that story that it didn't even feel like mine. It was only after we'd hung up, and I came back into the present moment, that the feelings came rushing back, and I realized that my pulse was racing, my heart was in my throat, and I was heavy with a distinct air of regret.

Oh shit, I thought. *I just told this guy stuff I haven't told anyone except Dr. Miller, and I'm not even sure exactly what I said.*

I spent hours agonizing, and I thought about emailing him and begging to take it all back. I even drafted an actual email: "I so respect all that you do in journalism, and I bet the answer is no, but is there any way that last answer can be off the record? I'm just not ready for my story to be in the world." But something stopped me from sending it.

Still, for the next several nights I lay awake in bed, racking my brain, trying to remember what I told the guy, but only turning up scraps of certain phrases ("an increase in patients, and really sick ones") and examples ("falling asleep after work, every day"). My biggest worry was that I'd said something I wouldn't want a patient to read about me, something that would make them lose faith in me. That's always my first thought in situations when I self-disclose publicly: *What would a patient think?*

Though much of what I've experienced and thought is publicly available, until that interview I had always been particular about how I presented myself in public: Anything I revealed about myself in my writing was the result of a conscious decision signaling that I was okay with people knowing that bit of personal information. My decision to write about my taking medication for a national magazine, for instance, came after significant reflection, nearly a year of distance from the X conversations that prompted it, and in-depth conversations with Dr. Miller. I knew I didn't want to tell people I was on medication just to tell people. I owed no one my history, but I wanted it to do more by writing something and examine the why. How someone who spends all day prescribing medications to healthcare workers can still stigmatize themselves for it. And if I do, what that means for other people and how hard it really is to fight the stigma and get help. Still, though I'm always aware that my patients can see whatever I write or say or tweet online, I also secretly hope they won't.

I also worry that certain things I say—about wanting to change the system or wishing medicine could be another way—might anger the university I work for and, technically, represent. I am acutely aware that when I talk about the burnout I and my healthcare patients are experiencing, the powers that be and the people reading this might interpret that as a criticism of my workplace. In truth, I believe that what my patients are experiencing—what we are all experiencing—is more the result of universal shortcomings in healthcare. For example, the fact that Luke's colleagues or supervisors don't know how to deal with his mental health struggles isn't the particular fault of his program, or his hospital. Looking at depression rates in doctors-in-training across all residency programs, we see there are no differences based on where residents train or what they study. The experience of residency itself is the stressor.[1]

None of what I discuss is intended to blame where I work, or where my patients do, because our work isn't solely to blame—the entire system of healthcare is. That system existed long before COVID, but COVID made its shortcomings painfully clear. Maybe that's why I never wrote to that reporter begging him to expunge my words from the record.

And in fact, he used what I said as the lede in the story. Now, everyone knows my secret. Knows that even psychiatrists are human.

But when I recount the incident to Dr. Miller—luckily, the next day is Therapy Thursday—I'm still agonizing. She listens intently, as she always does, then, looking directly at me, she says, "What worries you the most about having your story out there?"

Without hesitation, I respond, "I worry about what my patients will think. I always do. But I'm also worried that I made it about me, instead of about Luke or Naya or Janet or Megan."

"But isn't it about you sometimes? Or, can't it be?"

I nod. "I think it *has* to be. Especially if I'm falling asleep through a session or so angry at the pile-up of emails in my inbox that I don't want to respond. It gets to the point where I don't have a choice."

"Sure, but does everything about you have to be in relation to patients, and to work? Couldn't you worry about you, for you?"

"That feels like a bit of a foreign concept. A lot of me is work-me." I laugh a little. "I don't get much egg white, remember?" I say, referring to her drawing session.

She smiles. "I know the feeling. And you might get angry at me for pushing this, but what do *you* need? There used to be a *you*-you, before there was a doctor-you."

"I think I need to find her again. And maybe I already am."

She nods, waits for a few seconds, and then adds, "How does that feel?"

"Uncomfortable, but somehow, also right."

We sit together in silence, and even though I have the urge to talk or fidget, I don't. I just sit, finally okay with not having the answer.

Acknowledgments

I WROTE AND finished a book. If you are reading this, that statement is true and real, and even a little scary. It may take a while for that to sink in, but I know I could not have done any of it at all without the enormous team of people in my corner. A thank-you seems small, and words not enough, but it's a start.

I would never have written this if my friend Lucy Kalanithi at the height of the pandemic didn't ask me if I ever wanted to write a book, and as I hemmed and hawed, she followed up by asking the overachiever-competitor in me the right question: "But would you be mad if someone else did?" Those few words lit a fire in me that was kindled further by Lucy, Gabrielle Glaser, and my internet adopted mother, Rana Awdish, who all helped me formulate my thoughts, write a query letter, get an agent, and virtually held my hand along the way.

That agent, Kristin Van Ogtrop, has been phenomenal (along with the entire team at Inkwell), not just in shepherding me through my very first book but also in dealing with my overly emotional aware insights and anxieties along the way. I knew when I first met KVO that we were a good fit because she asked what inspired me and about my feelings. Jackpot.

Together, we sold my book to the wonderful team at Simon Element, originally to Leah Trouwborst, who believed in me and what I cared about in a way that made me feel seen. She passed the large, emotionally weighted baton to Ronnie Alvarado, who has helped this first-time author write something that is not just coherent but also feels right. She has also honored my vulnerability and boundaries along the way, in ways I could only hope for and never expected. Paula Derrow has also supported me in editing throughout, with amazing suggestions to make me a better writer, and even doing a little mothering when I let the emotions of the experience get the best of me. I am lucky to have found her and to have in my corner. I am also grateful to the rest of the Simon Element team for bringing this book to life: Richard Rhorer, Laura Jarrett, Davina Mock, Patrick Sullivan, Jessie McNeil, Jessica Preeg, Stacy Reichgott, Alyssa diPierro, and Maria Espinosa. Thank you also to Elizabeth Shreve for helping people know about this book and me, and, also, to Brandie Thurman, who helped me format this when even the idea of spacing and endnotes burned me out, you helped more than you know.

My proposal did not initially include patient stories, but I am honored that it could. I do not for one day take my job for granted, nor the trust that is offered to me. To the patients I see every day and the people I interviewed whose stories make up the composites, thank you. I am who I am, and I care about what I do, because you have informed that passion in ways I couldn't even start to explain. I am grateful for the privilege of hearing your stories, and that includes all the patients I had in training and medical school who taught me how to be a psychiatrist.

To make sure my composites were truly honoring healthcare workers' experiences and were culturally sensitive, I had a few health-care-worker friends provide early reads and give feedback. To Rana, Lucy, Shoshana Ungerleider, Amanda Calhoun, Ashley Bartholomew, and Kiera Quinlan, thank you for the care you showed me and my work, and for making it better. Every comment you gave me was insightful, and I do not take your time for granted. I also am incredibly grateful to a few of my other more frequent hand-holders who are medical writers themselves, my "Big Sis" Jen Gunter, Pooja Lakshmin, Jack Turban, Chase Anderson, and Jessica Zucker, for somehow always knowing what to say (and not to say), and helping me feel less alone in an otherwise very isolating process.

Laura Norkin also read a draft, and she has been an instrumental figure in my writing development. I call you my "fairy god editor" because that is truly what you are. I am also thankful to the people who supported me as a writer from the beginning, reading my work and amplifying it, as well as replying to my shady DMs asking to write for them, in particular, Cindi Leive and Carolyn Kylstra.

To Kiana Azizian, Taylor Swift, Cleo Wade, Mary Oliver, Maggie Smith, Lily Allen, Mr. Rogers, and everyone else whose words I turn to when I struggle with my own—thank you for getting me, even when I don't even get myself.

I would also never have been able to get to this point at all if it were not for the people always in my corner:

To the not-yet-named friends who support me in everything I do; naming you all would be like writing my senior page, and I am sure I would forget someone and feel horrible about it, so I'm not going to list names (even though I know some of you probably were hoping to see your name in my book). I hope you know who you are, because I try to tell you how much you mean to me all the time. You are the people I text or send videos to when something happens, or when I'm just bored, that I have met in all stages of my life and places, and who I turn to when I need someone to listen to me rant, cry, laugh, or plan a vacation as a distraction. I am sure I would not have written a book, much less come out of all the stages of training and even this pandemic emotionally intact, without you. Thank you times a million.

To my mentors and teachers—like Mrs. Houston, who got me interested in science by getting me to chant about osmosis on the desk in seventh grade, and Sallie DeGolia, who helped me find my way in psychiatry by supporting my multitasking—thank you all for making science cool and helping this overachiever thrive. A special shout out to Kirsten Wilkins, for the mentorship, friendship, and big sisterhood. I know I would have left medical school if I didn't find you and psychiatry, and our mutual love of *Suri's Burn Book*. Thanks for not letting me drop out, and for supporting me in being me. Even if that means I sometimes have to do a 5K with you.

And to my family . . . how do you really thank someone for helping you to become who you are while still making sure you laugh along the way? I am not sure that is possible, but I promised the kids they would be mentioned somewhere, so here goes: To Steve, Katie, Cam, Nathaniel, Charlotte, and Whit, Kim, Dan, Jonah, Eli, and Ari, Kyle, and Lauren, thank you (all in your own ways) for the support, role modeling, advice, and fun. In other words, well, everything. The mountain was high, but it has been worth the climb. To Grandma Helene, who regularly tells me what I do is important, to Aunt Sondra, who helped me love books in the first place, and also to Aunt Hyla and Uncle Larry, for being around and supporting me with dinner, with a side of legal or writing advice, thank you.

And, of course, thank you to my mom and dad, for wanting a fourth kid and encouraging me to be myself, big feelings and all. Thank you for having my back, even when I got kicked out of class. I hope you know I learned from everything I went through and that you did a great job raising this overly emotional perfectionist, even if I had big shoes to fill. I promise not to use everything from my life as a story for everyone else. I love you.

Last but never least, to the real Dr. Miller, you know who you are, I look forward to processing this after you read it, for years to come. Thank you for helping me help others.

Notes

CHAPTER 2

1. L. N. Dyrbye, A. Eacker, S. J. Durning, et al., "The Impact of Stigma and Personal Experiences on the Help-Seeking Behaviors of Medical Students with Burnout," *Academic Medicine* 90, no. 7 (2015): 961–969, https://doi.org/10.1097/ACM.0000000000000655.

2. Ibid.

3. F. W. Hafferty and R. Franks, "The Hidden Curriculum, Ethics Teaching, and the Structure of Medical Education," *Academic Medicine* 69 (1994): 861–871.

4. C. P. West, L. N. Dyrbye, and T. D. Shanafelt, "Physician Burnout: Contributors, Consequences and Solutions," *Journal of Internal Medicine* 283, no. 6 (2018): 516–529.

5. D. A. Mata, M. A. Ramos, N. Bansal, et al., "Prevalence of Depression and Depressive Symptoms Among Resident Physicians: A Systematic Review and Meta-analysis," *JAMA* 314, no. 22 (December 8, 2015): 2373–2383, https://doi.org/10.1001/jama.2015.15845; PMID 26647259; PMCID: PMC4866499.

6. M. A. Davis, B. A. Y. Cher, C. R. Friese, et al., "Association of US Nurse and Physician Occupation with Risk of Suicide," *JAMA Psychiatry* 78, no. 6 (2021): 1–8, https://doi.org/10.1001/jamapsychiatry.2021.0154.

7. T. D. Shanafelt, L. N. Dyrbye, C. P. West, et al., "Suicidal Ideation and Attitudes Regarding Help Seeking in US Physicians Relative to the US Working Population," *Mayo Clinic Proceedings* 96, no. 8 (2021): 2067–2080, https://doi.org/10.1016/j.mayocp.2021.01.033.

8. Accreditation Council for Graduate Medical Education, ACGME Common Program Requirements (Residency), February 3, 2020, updated March 2022, https://www.acgme.org/globalassets/PFAssets /ProgramRequirements/CPRResidency_2022v2.pdf.

9. A. L. Aaronson, K. Backes, G. Agarwal, et al., "Mental Health During Residency Training: Assessing the Barriers to Seeking Care," *Academic Psychiatry* 42, no. 4 (2018): 469–472, https://doi.org/10.1007/s40596 -017-0881-3.

10. Kaiser Family Foundation, Washington Post Healthcare Workers Survey, https://www.kff.org/report-section/kff-the-washington-post -frontline-health-care-workers-survey-toll-of-the-pandemic.

11. C. Guille, H. Speller, R. Laff, et al., "Utilization and Barriers to Mental Health Services Among Depressed Medical Interns: A Prospective Multisite Study, *Journal of Graduate Medical Education* 2, no. 2 (2010): 210–214, https://doi.org/10.4300/JGME-D-09-00086.1.

12. Substance Abuse and Mental Health Services Administration, "Impact of the DSM-IV to DSM-5 Changes on the National Survey on Drug Use and Health," Table 3.13, DSM-IV to DSM-5 Obsessive-Compulsive Disorder Comparison, June 2016, https://www.ncbi.nlm.nih.gov /books/NBK519704/table/ch3.t13/.

13. C. Ferrando and C. Selai, "A Systematic Review and Meta-analysis on the Effectiveness of Exposure and Response Prevention Therapy in the Treatment of Obsessive-Compulsive Disorder," *Journal of Obsessive-Compulsive and Related Disorders* 31 (2021): 100684.

14. American Psychological Association, "Habituation," *Dictionary of Psychology*, 2023, https://dictionary.apa.org/habituation.

15. C. Pittenger and M. H. Bloch, "Pharmacological Treatment of Obsessive-Compulsive Disorder," *Psychiatric Clinics of North America* 37, no. 3 (2014): 375–391, https://doi.org/10.1016/j.psc.2014.05.006.

CHAPTER 3

1. Z. Di Blasi, E. Harkness, E. Ernst, et al., "Influence of Context Effects on Health Outcomes: A Systematic Review," *The Lancet* 357, no. 9258 (March 2001): 757–762.

2. A. B. Brooks, P. L. Herrmann, and S. Andreas, "The Use of Banter in Psychotherapy: A Systematic Literature Review," *Counseling and Psychotherapy Research* 21, no. 3 (September 2021): 570–586.

3. Di Blasi, Harkness, Ernst, et al., "Influence of Context Effects," 757–762.

4. R. Ruskin, I. Sakinofsky, R. M. Bagby, et al., "Impact of Patient Suicide on Psychiatrists and Psychiatric Trainees," *Academic Psychiatry* 28, no. 2 (2004): 104–110, https://doi.org/10.1176/appi.ap.28.2.104.

5. David Jones, "A few years ago I wrote a short poem," Tumblr, 2017, https://story-dj.tumblr.com/post/153014781868/a-few-years-ago-i-wrote-a-short-poem-that-went.

CHAPTER 4

1. A. S. Brett and C. W. Goodman, "First Impressions: Should We Include Race or Ethnicity at the Beginning of Clinical Case Presentations?," *New England Journal of Medicine* 385, no. 27 (2021): 2497–2499, https://doi.org/10.1056/NEJMp2112312.

2. J. A. Hayes, C. J. Gelso, and A. M. Hummel, "Managing Countertransference," *Psychotherapy* 48, no. 1 (2011): 88.

3. Ibid.

4. Carl Jung, letter to Kendig B. Cully, September 25, 1931, quoted in *Oxford Essential Quotations*, ed. Susan Ratcliffe (Oxford, UK: Oxford University Press, 2016.) https://www.oxfordreference.com/display/10.1093/acref/9780191826719.001.0001/q-oro-ed4-00006107.

5. M. Sun, T. Oliwa, M. E. Peek, et al., "Negative Patient Descriptors: Documenting Racial Bias in the Electronic Health Record," *Health Affairs (Millwood)* 41, no. 2 (2022): 203–211, https://doi.org/10.1377/hlthaff.2021.01423.

6. X. Zhang, M. Carabello, T. Hill, et al., "Trends of Racial/Ethnic Differences in Emergency Department Care Outcomes Among Adults in the United States From 2005 to 2016," *Frontiers in Medicine* (Lausanne) 7 (June 25, 2020): 300, https://doi.org/10.3389/fmed.2020.00300.

7. D. R. Williams and T. D. Rucker, "Understanding and Addressing Racial Disparities in Health Care," *Health Care Financing Review* 21, no. 4 (Summer 2000): 75–90, PMID 11481746; PMCID: PMC4194634.

8.   J. Groopman, "What's the Trouble? How Doctors Think," *The New Yorker*, January 21, 2007, https://www.newyorker.com/magazine/2007 /01/29/whats-the-trouble.

9.   J. C. Huffman, M. H. Pollack, and T. A. Stern, "Panic Disorder and Chest Pain: Mechanisms, Morbidity, and Management," *Primary Care Companion to Journal of Clinical Psychiatry* 4, no. 2 (April 2002): 54– 62, https://doi.org/10.4088/pcc.v04n0203; PMID 15014745; PMCID: PMC181226.

10. D. A. Barr, J. Matsui, S. F. Wanat, et al., "Chemistry Courses as the Turning Point for Premedical Students," *Advances in Health Sciences Education: Theory and Practice* 15, no. 1 (2010): 45–54, https://doi .org/10.1007/s10459-009-9165-3.

11. Association of American Medical Colleges, "Table A-16: MCAT Scores and GPAs for Applicants and Matriculants to U.S. MD-Granting Medical Schools 2018–2019 through 2022–2023", 2022, https://www .aamc.org/media/6056/download.

12. K. Lovecchio and L. Dundes, "Premed Survival: Understanding the Culling Process in Premedical Undergraduate Education," *Academic Medicine* 77, no. 7 (2002): 719–724, https://doi.org/10.1097/00001888 -200207000-00016.

13. Association of American Medical Colleges, Students and Residents, "The MCAT Exam Score Scale," 2023, https://students-residents.aamc .org/mcat-scores/mcat-exam-score-scale.

14. W. T. Basco Jr, G. E. Gilbert, A. W. Chessman, et al., "The Ability of a Medical School Admission Process to Predict Clinical Performance and Patients' Satisfaction," *Academic Medicine* 75, no. 7 (2000): 743– 747, https://doi.org/10.1097/00001888-200007000-00021.

15. Association of American Medical Colleges, "2021 Facts: Applicants and Matriculants Data," https://www.aamc.org/data-reports/students -residents/interactive-data/2021-facts-applicants-and-matriculants -data.

16. M. S. Barrett and J. S. Berman, "Is Psychotherapy More Effective When Therapists Disclose Information About Themselves?," *Journal of Consulting and Clinical Psychology* 69, no. 4 (2001): 597–603, https://doi .org/10.1037/0022-006X.69.4.597.

CHAPTER 5

1. S. Ganesan, M. Magee, J. E. Stone, et al., "The Impact of Shift Work on Sleep, Alertness and Performance in Healthcare Workers," *Scientific Reports* 9, no. 1 (March 15, 2019): 4635, https://doi.org/10.1038/s41598-019-40914-x.

2. S. E. Merel, C. M. McKinney, P. Ufkes, et al., "Sitting at Patients' Bedsides May Improve Patients' Perceptions of Physician Communication Skills," *Journal of Hospital Medicine* 11, no. 12 (2016): 865–868, https://doi.org/10.1002/jhm.2634.

3. J. V. Silva and I. Carvalho, "Physicians Experiencing Intense Emotions While Seeing Their Patients: What Happens?," *Permanente Journal* 20, no. 3 (2016): 15-229, https://doi.org/10.7812/TPP/15-229.

4. M. Neumann, F. Edelhäuser, D. Tauschel, et al., "Empathy Decline and Its Reasons: A Systematic Review of Studies with Medical Students and Residents, *Academic Medicine* 86, no. 8 (2011): 996–1009, https://doi.org/10.1097/ACM.0b013e318221e615.

5. K. Doulougeri, E. Panagopoulou, and A. Montgomery, "(How) Do Medical Students Regulate Their Emotions?," *BMC Medical Education* 16, no. 1 (December 12, 2016): 312, https://doi.org/10.1186/s12909-016-0832-9.

6. A. Kerasidou and R. Horn, "Making Space for Empathy: Supporting Doctors in the Emotional Labour of Clinical Care," *BMC Medical Ethics* 17 (January 27, 2016): 8, https://doi.org/10.1186/s12910-016-0091-7.

7. P. Croskerry, A. Abbass, and A. W. Wu, "Emotional Influences in Patient Safety," *Journal of Patient Safety* 6, no. 4 (2010): 199–205, https://doi.org/10.1097/pts.0b013e3181f6c01a.

8. J. V. Silva and I. Carvalho, "Physicians Experiencing Intense Emotions."

9. P. Sullivan, "What's Sewn In," *Canadian Family Physician* 62, no. 5 (May 2016): 422–423, PMID 27255626; PMCID: PMC4865343.

10. World Health Organization, "Burnout as an 'Occupational Phenomenon': International Classification of Diseases," May 18, 2019, https://www.who.int/news/item/28-05-2019-burn-out-an-occupational-phenomenon-international-classification-of-diseases; T. D. Shanafelt, S. Boone, L. Tan, et al., "Burnout and Satisfaction with Work-Life Bal-

ance Among US Physicians Relative to the General US Population," *Archives of Internal Medicine* 172 (2012): 1377–1385.

11. T. D. Shanafelt, C. Sinsky, L. N. Dyrbye, et al., "Burnout Among Physicians Compared with Individuals with a Professional or Doctoral Degree in a Field Outside of Medicine," *Mayo Clinic Proceedings* 94, no. 3 (March 1, 2019): 549–551.

12. G. Jackson-Koku and P. Grime, "Emotion Regulation and Burnout in Doctors: A Systematic Review," *Occupational Medicine* 69, no. 1 (January 2019): 9–21.

13. L. N. Dyrbye, M. R. Thomas, F. S. Massie, et al., "Burnout and Suicidal Ideation Among US Medical Students," *Annals of Internal Medicine* 149, no. 5 (September 2, 2008): 334–341.

14. A. S. L. Knol, T. Koole, M. Desmet, et al., "How Speakers Orient to the Notable Absence of Talk: A Conversation Analytic Perspective on Silence in Psychodynamic Therapy," *Frontiers in Psychology* 11 (December 7, 2020): 584927, https://doi.org/10.3389/fpsyg.2020.584927.

15. R. Valle, "Toward a Psychology of Silence," *Humanistic Psychologist* 47, no. 3 (2019): 219–261, https://doi.org/10.1037/hum0000120.

16. A. Salles and J. Gold, "Health Care Workers Aren't Just Heroes. We're Also Scared and Exposed," *Vox*, April 2, 2020, https://www.vox.com/2020/4/2/21204402/coronavirus-covid-19-doctors-nurses-health-care-workers.

CHAPTER 6

1. A. L. Baier, A. C. Kline, and N. C. Feeny, "Therapeutic Alliance as a Mediator of Change: A Systematic Review and Evaluation of Research," *Clinical Psychology Review* 82 (2020): 101921; C. Flückiger, A. C. Del Re, B. E. Wampold, et al., "The Alliance in Adult Psychotherapy: A Meta-analytic Synthesis," *Psychotherapy* 55, no. 4 (2018): 316–340, https://doi.org/10.1037/pst0000172.

2. Rotger J. Mercadal and V. Cabré, "Therapeutic Alliance in Online and Face-to-face Psychological Treatment: Comparative Study," *Journal of Medical Internet Research, Mental Health* 9, no. 5 (2022): e36775.

CHAPTER 7

1. C. Vindrola-Padros, L. Andrews, A. Dowrick, et al., "Perceptions and Experiences of Healthcare Workers During the COVID-19 Pandemic in the UK," *BMJ Open* 10, no. 11 (2020): e040503.

2. C. Lebel, A. MacKinnon, M. Bagshawe, et al., "Elevated Depression and Anxiety Symptoms Among Pregnant Individuals During the COVID-19 Pandemic," *Journal of Affective Disorders* 277 (December 1, 2020): 5–13, https://doi.org/10.1016/j.jad.2020.07.126; erratum in 279 (January 15, 2021): 377–379; PMID 32777604; PMCID: PMC7395614.

3. C. X. W. Zhang, J. C. Okeke, R. D. Levitan, et al., "Evaluating Depression and Anxiety Throughout Pregnancy and After Birth: Impact of the COVID-19 Pandemic," *American Journal of Obstetrics and Gynecology* 4, no. 3 (2022): 100605, https://doi.org/10.1016/j.ajogmf.2022.100605.

4. E. Frank, Z. Zhao, Y. Fang, et al., "Experiences of Work-Family Conflict and Mental Health Symptoms by Gender Among Physician Parents During the COVID-19 Pandemic," *JAMA Network Open* 4, no. 11 (2021): e2134315, https://doi.org/10.1001/jamanetworkopen.2021.34315.

5. F. Hossain and A. Clatty, "Self-care Strategies in Response to Nurses' Moral Injury During COVID-19 Pandemic," *Nursing Ethics* 28, no. 1 (2021): 23–32, https://doi.org/10.1177/0969733020961825.

6. J. A. Nieuwsma, E. C. O'Brien, H. Xu, et al., "Patterns of Potential Moral Injury in Post-9/11 Combat Veterans and COVID-19 Healthcare Workers," *Journal of General Internal Medicine* 37, no. 8 (2022): 2033–2040, https://doi.org/10.1007/s11606-022-07487-4.

7. V. Williamson, S. A. M. Stevelink, and N. Greenberg, "Occupational Moral Injury and Mental Health: Systematic Review and Meta-Analysis," *British Journal of Psychiatry* 212, no. 6 (June 2018): 339–346, https://www.doi.org10.1192/bjp.2018.55; PMID 29786495.

8. M. Roycroft, D. Wilkes, S. Pattani, et al., "Limiting Moral Injury in Healthcare Professionals During the COVID-19 Pandemic," *Occupational Medicine* (London) 70, no. 5 (July 17, 2020): 312–314, https://doi.org/10.1093/occmed/kqaa087; PMID 32428213; PMCID: PMC7313795.

CHAPTER 9

1. L. G. Öst, A. Havnen, B. Hansen, et al., "Cognitive Behavioral Treatments of Obsessive-Compulsive Disorder: A Systematic Review and Meta-analysis of Studies Published 1993–2014," *Clinical Psychology Review* 40 (2015): 156–169, https://doi.org/10.1016/j.cpr.2015.06.003.

2. L. C. Kaldjian, L. A. Shinkunas, H. S. Reisinger, et al., "Attitudes About Sickness Presenteeism in Medical Training: Is There a Hidden Curriculum?," *Antimicrobial Resistance & Infection Control* 8, no. 1 (December 2019): 1–9.

3. A. B. Schultz, C. Y. Chen, and D. W. Edington, "The Cost and Impact of Health Conditions on Presenteeism to Employers: A Review of the Literature," *Pharmacoeconomics* 27, no. 5 (2009): 365–378, https://doi.org/10.2165/00019053-200927050-00002.

4. P. Pei, G. Lin, G. Li, et al., "The Association Between Doctors' Presenteeism and Job Burnout: A Cross-sectional Survey Study in China," *BMC Health Services Research* 20, no. 1 (2020): 1–7.

5. J. E. Szymczak, S. Smathers, C. Hoegg, et al., "Reasons Why Physicians and Advanced Practice Clinicians Work While Sick: A Mixed-Methods Analysis," *JAMA Pediatrics* 169, no. 9 (2015): 815–821, https://doi.org/10.1001/jamapediatrics.2015.0684.

6. L. C. Kaldjian, L. A. Shinkunas, H. S. Reisinger, et al., "Attitudes About Sickness Presenteeism in Medical Training: Is There a Hidden Curriculum?," *Antimicrobial Resistance & Infection Control* 8 (2019): 149, https://doi.org/10.1186/s13756-019-0602-7.

7. S. B. Mossad, A. Deshpande, S. Schramm, et al., "Working Despite Having Influenza-Like Illness: Results of an Anonymous Survey of Healthcare Providers Who Care for Transplant Recipients," *Infection Control & Hospital Epidemiology* 38, no. 89 (2017): 966–969, https://doi.org/10.1017/ice.2017.91.

8. C. P. West, L. N. Dyrbye, C. Sinsky, et al., "Resilience and Burnout Among Physicians and the General US Working Population," *JAMA Network Open* 3, no. 7 (2020): e209385, https://doi.org/10.1001/jamanetworkopen.2020.9385.

9. Accreditation Council for Graduate Medical Education, "ACGME

Releases Revised Common Program Requirements, Section VI, The Learning and Working Environment Standards Reinforce Culture of Patient Safety and Physician Well-Being," March 10, 2017, https://www .acgme.org/globalassets/PDFs/Nasca-Community/ACGME-Common -Press-Release-3-10-2017.pdf.

10. A. B. Blum, F. Raiszadeh, S. Shea, et al., "US Public Opinion Regarding Proposed Limits on Resident Physician Work Hours," *BMC Medicine* 8 (June 1, 2010): 33, https://doi.org/10.1186/1741-7015-8-33; PMID 20515479; PMCID: PMC2901227.

11. L. Rosenbaum and D. Lamas, "Residents' Duty Hours—Toward an Empirical Narrative," *New England Journal of Medicine* 367, no. 21 (November 22, 2012): 2044–2049.

12. A. M. Williamson and A. Feyer, "Moderate Sleep Deprivation Produces Impairments in Cognitive and Motor Performance Equivalent to Legally Prescribed Levels of Alcohol Intoxication," *Occupational and Environmental Medicine* 57 (2000): 649–655.

13. A. B. Jena, M. Farid, D. Blumenthal, et al., "Association of Residency Work Hour Reform with Long Term Quality and Costs of Care of US Physicians: Observational Study," *BMJ* 366 (2019): l4134, https://doi .org/10.1136/bmj.l4134

14. L. K. Barger, M. D. Weaver, J. P. Sullivan, et al., "Impact of Work Schedules of Senior Resident Physicians on Patient and Resident Physician Safety: Nationwide, Prospective Cohort Study," *BMJ Medicine* 2, no. 1 (March 2023).

15. T. Nasca, "What New Resident Work Hours Mean for Physician Well-Being and Patient Safety," Health Affairs Forefront. February 9, 2017, https://www.healthaffairs.org/do/10.1377/forefront.20170209.05 8687.

16. K. L. Martin, "Residents Salary and Debt Report, 2020," Medscape, August 7, 2020, https://www.medscape.com/slideshow/2020-residents -salary-debt-report-6013072?faf=1#1.

17. M. Hanson, "Average Medical School Debt," Education Data Initiative, September 17, 2023, https://educationdata.org/average-medical -school-debt.

CHAPTER 11

1. University of Michigan Behavioral Health Workforce Research Center, "Estimating the Distribution of the U.S. Psychiatric Subspecialist Workforce," 2018, https://behavioralhealthworkforce.org/wp-content/uploads/2019/02/Y3-FA2-P2-Psych-Sub_Full-Report-FINAL2.19.2019.pdf.

2. A. F. Cook, V. M. Arora, K. A. Rasinski, et al., "The Prevalence of Medical Student Mistreatment and Its Association with Burnout," *Academic Medicine* 89, no. 5 (May 2014): 749–754, https://doi.org/10.1097/ACM.0000000000000204; PMID 24667503; PMCID: PMC4401419.

3. M. Trockel, C. Sinsky, C. P. West, et al., "Self-Valuation Challenges in the Culture and Practice of Medicine and Physician Well-Being," *Mayo Clinic Proceedings* 96, no. 8 (2021): 2123–2132, https://doi.org/10.1016/j.mayocp.2020.12.032.

4. K. D. Neff, M. C. Knox, P. Long, et al., "Caring for Others Without Losing Yourself: An Adaptation of the Mindful Self-Compassion Program for Healthcare Communities," *Journal of Clinical Psychology* 76, no. 9 (2020): 1543–1562, https://doi.org/10.1002/jclp.23007.

CHAPTER 12

1. M. Peters and J. King, "Perfectionism in Doctors," *BMJ* 16 (March 2012): 344.

2. C. Munro, "Simone Biles' Bravery Is a Lesson in Leadership for Everyone: It Takes More Courage to Step Back Than to Step Up," *The BMJ Opinion*, July 30, 2021, https://blogs.bmj.com/bmj/2021/07/30/simone-biles-bravery-is-a-lesson-in-leadership-for-everyone-it-takes-more-courage-to-step-back-than-to-step-up/.

3. M. B. Edmond, J. L. Deschenes, M. Eckler, et al., "Racial Bias in Using USMLE Step 1 Scores to Grant Internal Medicine Residency Interviews," *Academic Medicine* 76, no. 12 (2001): 1253–1256, https://doi.org/10.1097/00001888-200112000-00021.

4. L. Spring, D. Robillard, L. Gehlbach, et al., "Impact of Pass/Fail Grading on Medical Students' Well-Being and Academic Outcomes," *Medi-*

cal Education 45, no. 9 (2011): 867–877, https://doi.org/10.1111/j.1365 -2923.2011.03989.x; R. A. Bloodgood, J. G. Short, J. M. Jackson, et al., "A Change to Pass/Fail Grading in the First Two Years at One Medical School Results in Improved Psychological Well-Being," *Academic Medicine* 84, no. 5 (2009): 655–662, https://doi.org/10.1097 /ACM.0b013e31819f6d78.

5. D. B. Morris, P. A. Gruppuso, H. A. McGee, et al., "Diversity of the National Medical Student Body—Four Decades of Inequities," *New England Journal of Medicine* 384, no. 17 (2021): 1661–1668, https://doi .org/10.1056/NEJMsr2028487

6. L. O. O'Malley. "Addressing the Lack of Black Mental Health Professionals," *Insight into Diversity*, November 17, 2021, https://www .insightintodiversity.com/addressing-the-lack-of-black-mental-health -professionals.

7. S. G. Hofmann and D. E. Hinton, "Cross-cultural Aspects of Anxiety Disorders," *Current Psychiatry Reports* 16, no. 6 (June 2014): 450, https://doi.org/10.1007/s11920-014-0450-3; PMID 24744049; PMCID: PMC4037698.

8. D. Hamachek, "Psychodynamics of Normal and Neurotic Perfectionism," *Psychology* 15 (1978): 27–33.

9. K. S. Hu, J. T. Chibnall, and S. J. Slavin, "Maladaptive Perfectionism, Impostorism, and Cognitive Distortions: Threats to the Mental Health of Pre-clinical Medical Students," *Academic Psychiatry* 43, no. 4 (2019): 381–385, https://doi.org/10.1007/s40596-019-01031-z.

10. L. S. Rotenstein, M. A. Ramos, M. Torre, et al., "Prevalence of Depression, Depressive Symptoms, and Suicidal Ideation Among Medical Students: A Systematic Review and Meta-Analysis," *JAMA* 316, no. 21 (2016): 2214–2236, https://doi.org/10.1001/jama.2016.17324.

11. "Major Depression," National Institute of Mental Health, July 2023, https://www.nimh.nih.gov/health/statistics/major-depression.

12. M. K. Grace, "Depressive Symptoms, Burnout, and Declining Medical Career Interest Among Undergraduate Pre-medical Students," *International Journal of Medical Education* 9 (November 26, 2018): 302–308, https://doi.org/10.5116/ijme.5be5.8131.

13. M. Bateson, B. Brilot, and D. Nettle, "Anxiety: An Evolutionary Approach," *Canadian Journal of Psychiatry* 56, no. 12 (December 2011): 707–715.

14. N. M. Batelaan, R. C. Bosman, A. Muntingh, et al., "Risk of Relapse After Antidepressant Discontinuation in Anxiety Disorders, Obsessive-Compulsive Disorder, and Post-Traumatic Stress Disorder: Systematic Review and Meta-analysis of Relapse Prevention Trials," *BMJ* 358 (2017): j3927, https://doi.org/10.1136/bmj.j3927.

15. O. A. Almohammed, A. A. Alsalem, A. A. Almangour, et al., "Antidepressants and Health-Related Quality of Life (HRQoL) for Patients with Depression: Analysis of the Medical Expenditure Panel Survey from the United States," *PLOS One* 17, no. 4 (April 2022): e0265928.

CHAPTER 14

1. M. H. Imran, Z. Zhai, and M. Iqbal, "The Role of Religious Coping to Overcome Mental Distress and Anxiety During the COVID-19 Pandemic: An Integrative Review," *Analyses of Social Issues and Public* 22, no. 3, December 2022: 817–835.

2. S. K. Chow, B. Francis, Y. H. Ng, et al., "Religious Coping, Depression and Anxiety Among Healthcare Workers During the COVID-19 Pandemic: A Malaysian Perspective," *Healthcare* (Basel) 9, no. 1 (January 15, 2021): 79, https://doi.org/10.3390/healthcare9010079; PMID 33467744; PMCID: PMC7831030.

3. J. Kwak, S. Rajagopal, G. Handzo, et al., "Perspectives of Board-Certified Healthcare Chaplains on Challenges and Adaptations in Delivery of Spiritual Care in the COVID-19 Era: Findings from an Online Survey," *Palliative Medicine* 36, no. 1 (January 2022): 105–113.

4. M. H. Rasmussen, M. Strøm, J. Wohlfahrt, et al., "Risk, Treatment Duration, and Recurrence Risk of Postpartum Affective Disorder in Women with No Prior Psychiatric History: A Population-Based Cohort Study." *PLOS Medicine* 14, no. 9 (September 26, 2017): e1002392, https://doi.org/10.1371/journal.pmed.1002392.

5. C. Benjet, E. Bromet, E. G. Karam, et al., "The Epidemiology of Trau-

matic Event Exposure Worldwide: Results from the World Mental Health Survey Consortium." *Psychological Medicine* 46, no. 2 (January 2016): 327–343. https://doi.org/10.1017/S0033291715001981; PMID: 26511595; PMCID: PMC4869975.

6. U.S. Department of Veterans Affairs, PTSD: National Center for PTSD, "How Common Is PTSD in Adults?" February 3, 2023, https://www .ptsd.va.gov/understand/common/common_adults.asp.

7. American Psychiatric Association, "What Is Posttraumatic Stress Disorder (PTSD)," November 2022, https://www.psychiatry.org /patients-families/ptsd/what-is-ptsd.

8. T. Rodney, O. Heidari, H. N. Miller, et al., "Posttraumatic Stress Disorder in Nurses in the United States: Prevalence and Effect on Role," *Journal of Nursing Management* 30, no. 1 (2022): 226–233, https://doi .org/10.1111/jonm.13478.

9. J. D. Flory and R. Yehuda, "Comorbidity Between Post-Traumatic Stress Disorder and Major Depressive Disorder: Alternative Explanations and Treatment Considerations," *Dialogues in Clinical Neuroscience* 71, no. 2 (June 2015): 141–150, https://doi.org/ 10.31887 /DCNS.2015.17.2/jflory; PMID 26246789; PMCID: PMC4518698.

10. *New York Times* staff, "An Incalculable Loss," *New York Times*, May 27, 2020, https://www.nytimes.com/interactive/2020/05/24/us/us-corona virus-deaths-100000.html.

CHAPTER 15

1. P. Grossman, L. Niemann, S. Schmidt, et al., "Mindfulness-based Stress Reduction and Health Benefits: A Meta-analysis," *Journal of Psychosomatic Research* 57, no. 1 (July 2004): 35–43.

CHAPTER 17

1. K. Baikie and K. Wilhelm, "Emotional and Physical Health Benefits of Expressive Writing," *Advances in Psychiatric Treatment* 11, no. 5 (2005): 338–346, https://doi.org/10.1192/apt.11.5.338.

2. A. A. Green and E. V. Kinchen, "The Effects of Mindfulness Medita-
    tion on Stress and Burnout in Nurses," *Journal of Holistic Nursing* 39,
    no. 4 (2021): 356–368, https://doi.org/10.1177/08980101211015818;
    E. H. Morrow, T. Mai, B. Choi, et al., "Comparison of Mindful-
    ness Interventions for Healthcare Professionals: A Mixed-Methods
    Study," *Complementary Therapies in Medicine* 70 (November 1, 2022):
    102864.

3. J. B. Luoma, C. E. Martin, and J. L. Pearson, "Contact with Mental
    Health and Primary Care Providers Before Suicide: A Review of the
    Evidence," *American Journal of Psychiatry* 159 (2002): 909–916.

4. M. A. Graber, G. Bergus, J. D. Dawson, et al., "Effect of a Patient's Psychi-
    atric History on Physicians' Estimation of Probability of Disease," *Jour-
    nal of General Internal Medicine* 15, no. 3 (March 2000): 204–206, https://
    doi.org/10.1046/j.1525-1497.2000.04399.x; PMID 10718903; PMCID:
    PMC1495355.

5. A. Fiorillo and N. Sartorius, "Mortality Gap and Physical Comorbid-
    ity of People with Severe Mental Disorders: The Public Health Scan-
    dal," *Annals of General Psychiatry* 20, no. 52 (2021): n.p., https://doi
    .org/10.1186/s12991-021-00374-y.

CHAPTER 18

1. A. J. Milam, O. Oboh, Z. Brown, et al., "Symptoms of Depression and
    Anxiety Among Black Medical Students: The Role of Peer Connect-
    edness and Perceived Discrimination," *Journal of Racial Ethnic Health
    Disparities* 9, no. 6 (2022): 2180–2187, https://doi.org/10.1007/s40615
    -021-01157-7.

2. M. Pheister, R. M. Peters, and M. I. Wrzosek, "The Impact of Mental
    Illness Disclosure in Applying for Residency," *Academic Psychiatry* 44,
    no. 5 (2020): 554–561, https://doi.org/10.1007/s40596-020-01227-8.

3. L. M. Meeks, B. Case, K. Herzer, et al., "Change in Prevalence of Disabil-
    ities and Accommodation Practices Among US Medical Schools, 2016
    vs 2019," *JAMA* 322, no. 20 (2019): 2022–2024, https://doi.org/10.1001
    /jama.2019.15372.

4. L. M. Meeks, M. Plegue, B. Case, et al., "Assessment of Disclosure of

Psychological Disability Among US Medical Students," *JAMA Network Open* 3, no. 7 (2020): e2011165, https://doi.org/10.1001/jamanetwork open.2020.11165.

5. K. Woolf, J. Cave, I. C. McManus, et al., "'It Gives You an Understanding You Can't Get from Any Book': The Relationship Between Medical Students' and Doctors' Personal Illness Experiences and Their Performance: A Qualitative and Quantitative Study," *BMC Medical Education* 7, no. 1 (December 2007): 1–8.

6. M. Friedrich, "Depression Is the Leading Cause of Disability Around the World," *JAMA* 317, no. 15 (2017): 1517, https://doi.org/10.1001 /jama.2017.3826.

7. Healthy Minds Network, "Healthy Minds Study among Colleges and Universities, year [2021–22]," Healthy Minds Network, University of Michigan, University of California Los Angeles, Boston University, and Wayne State University, https://healthymindsnetwork.org /research/data-for-researchers.

8. S. K. Lipson, A. Kern, D. Eisenberg, et al., "Mental Health Disparities Among College Students of Color," *Journal of Adolescent Health* 63, no. 3 (2018): 348–356, https://doi.org/10.1016/j.jadohealth.2018.04.014.

9. L. N. Dyrbye, C. P. West, C. A. Sinsky, et al., "Medical Licensure Questions and Physician Reluctance to Seek Care for Mental Health Conditions," *Mayo Clinic Proceedings* 92, no. 10 (2017): 1486–1493. https: //doi.org/10.1016/j.mayocp.2017.06.020.

10. D. Saddawi-Konefka, A. Brown, I. Eisenhart, et al., "Consistency Between State Medical License Applications and Recommendations Regarding Physician Mental Health," *JAMA* 325, no. 19 (2021): 2017–2018, https://doi.org/10.1001/jama.2021.2275.

11. L. N. Dyrbye, C. P. West, C. A. Sinsky, et al., "Medical Licensure Questions and Physician Reluctance to Seek Care for Mental Health Conditions," *Mayo Clinic Proceedings* 92, no. 10 (2017): 1486–1493, https: //doi.org/10.1016/j.mayocp.2017.06.020.

12. M. J. Halter, D. G. Rolin, M. Adamaszek, et al., "State Nursing Licensure Questions about Mental Illness and Compliance with the Americans with Disabilities Act," *Journal of Psychosocial Nursing and Mental Health Services* 57, no. 8 (August 1, 2019): 17–22, https://doi

.org/10.3928/02793695-20190405-02; J. E. Boyd, B. Graunke, F. J. Frese, et al., "State Psychology Licensure Questions about Mental Illness and Compliance with the Americans with Disabilities Act,"*American Journal of Orthopsychiatry* 86, no 6 (2016): 620–631. https://doi .org/10.1037/ort0000177.

13. M. Gabriel and V. Sharma, "Antidepressant Discontinuation Syndrome," *Canadian Medical Association Journal* 189, no. 21 (May 29, 2017): e747, https://doi.org/10.1503/cmaj.160991; PMID 28554948; PMCID: PMC5449237.

14. National Institutes of Health: National Institute on Drug Abuse, "Drugs Brains, and Behavior: The Science of Addiction, Drug Misuse and Addiction," July 2020, https://nida.nih.gov/publications/drugs-brains -behavior-science-addiction/drug-misuse-addiction.

CHAPTER 19

1. A. M. Hoffman and J. Kaire, "Comfortably Numb: Effects of Prolonged Media Coverage," *Journal of Conflict Resolution* 64, no. 9 (2020): 1666–1692, https://doi.org/10.1177/0022002720907675.

2. J. A. Gold, "No, You Shouldn't Call Someone 'Crazy.' But Do We Have To Ban The Word Entirely?" *Self*, November 27, 2019, https://www.self .com/story/crazy-mental-health-stigma.

3. M. W. Gallagher, L. J. Long, and C. A. Phillips, "Hope, Optimism, Self-efficacy, and Posttraumatic Stress Disorder: A Meta-analytic Review of the Protective Effects of Positive Expectancies," *Journal of Clinical Psychology* 76, no. 3 (2020): 329–355, https://doi.org/10.1002 /jclp.22882.

4. F. B. Bryant and J. A. Cvengros, "Distinguishing Hope and Optimism: Two Sides of a Coin, or Two Separate Coins?," *Journal of Social and Clinical Psychology* 23, no. 2 (2004): 273–302, https://https://doi .org/10.1521/jscp.23.2.273.31018.

5. R. J. Reichard, J. B. Avey, S. Lopez, et al., "Having the Will and Finding the Way: A Review and Meta-analysis of Hope at Work," *Journal of Positive Psychology* 8, no. 4 (July 1, 2013): 292–304.

6. Positive Psychology Center, "Adult Hope Scale," 2023, https://ppc.sas .upenn.edu/resources/questionnaires-researchers/adult-hope-scale.

7. L. Day, K. Hanson, J. Maltby, et al., "Hope Uniquely Predicts Objective Academic Achievement Above Intelligence, Personality, and Previous Academic Achievement," *Journal of Research in Personality* 44, no. 4 (August 1, 2010): 550–553.

8. K. L. Wolfe, P. A. Nakonezny, V. J. Owen, et al., "Hopelessness as a Predictor of Suicide Ideation in Depressed Male and Female Adolescent Youth," *Suicide and Life-Threatening Behavior* 49, no. 1 (February 2019): 253–263, https://doi.org/10.1111/sltb.12428; PMID 29267993; PMCID: PMC6013307.

9. T. Dazzi, R. Gribble, S. Wessely, et al., "Does Asking About Suicide and Related Behaviours Induce Suicidal Ideation? What Is the Evidence?," *Psychological Medicine* 44, no. 16 (2014): 3361–3363, https: //doi.org/10.1017/S0033291714001299.

10. S. Stierwalt, "Why Do Smells Trigger Memories?," *Scientific American*, June 29, 2020, https://www.scientificamerican.com/article/why-do -smells-trigger-memories1/.

11. American Association of Colleges of Nursing, "Nursing Shortage Fact Sheet, October 2022," https://www.aacnnursing.org/news-information /fact-sheets/nursing-shortage.

12. M. K. Shah, N. Gandrakota, J. P. Cimiotti, et al., "Prevalence of and Factors Associated with Nurse Burnout in the US," *JAMA Network Open* 4, no. 2 (February 1, 2021) e2036469, https://doi.org/10.1001/jamanetwork open.2020.36469; erratum in 4, no. 3 (March 1, 2021): e215373; PMID 33538823; PMCID: PMC7862989.

13. American Nurses Association, "COVID-19 Impact Assessment Survey," March 1, 2022, https://www.nursingworld.org/~4a2260 /contentassets/872ebb13c63f44f6b11a1bd0c74907c9/covid-19-two -year-impact-assessment-written-report-final.pdf.

14. L. H. Aiken, S. P. Clarke, D. M. Sloane, et al., "Hospital Nurse Staffing and Patient Mortality, Nurse Burnout, and Job Dissatisfaction," *JAMA* 288, no. 16 (2002): 1987–1993, https:// doi.org/10.1001 /jama.288.16.1987.

15. M. Brenan, "Nurses Retain Top Ethics Rating in U.S., but Below 2020 High," *Gallup*, January 10, 2023, https://news.gallup.com/poll/467804 /nurses-retain-top-ethics-rating-below-2020-high.aspx.

16. L. E. Watkins, K. R. Sprang, and B. O. Rothbaum, "Treating PTSD: A Review of Evidence-Based Psychotherapy Interventions," *Frontiers in Behavioral Neuroscience* 12 (November 2, 2018): 258, https: //doi.org/10.3389/fnbeh.2018.00258. PMID 30450043; PMCID: PMC 6224348.

17. J. D. Flory and R. Yehuda, "Comorbidity Between Post-traumatic Stress Disorder and Major Depressive Disorder: Alternative Explanations and Treatment Considerations," *Dialogues in Clinical Neuroscience* 17, no. 2 (June 2015): 141–150, https://doi.org/10.31887/DCNS.2015.17.2 /jflory; PMID 26246789; PMCID: PMC4518698.

CHAPTER 20

1. T. D. Shanafelt, K. L. Kaups, H. Nelson, et al., "An Interactive Individualized Intervention to Promote Behavioral Change to Increase Personal Well-Being in US Surgeons," *Annals of Surgery* 259, no. 1 (2014): 82–88, https://doi.org/10.1097/SLA.0b013e3182a58fa4.

2. R. N. Remen, *Kitchen Table Wisdom: Stories That Heal* (New York: Riverhead Books, 2006).

CHAPTER 22

1. D. P. Edelson, B. Litzinger, V. Arora, et al., "Improving In-Hospital Cardiac Arrest Process and Outcomes With Performance Debriefing," *Archives of Internal Medicine* 168, no. 10 (2008): 1063–1069, https://doi .org/10.1001/archinte.168.10.1063.

2. S. Kapoor, C. K. Morgan, M. A. Siddique, et al., "'Sacred Pause' in the ICU: Evaluation of a Ritual and Intervention to Lower Distress and Burnout," *American Journal of Hospital Palliative Care* 35, no. 10 (2018): 1337–1341, https://doi.org/10.1177/1049909118768247.

3. L. N. Dyrbye, B. Major-Elechi, J. T. Hays, et al., "Relationship Between Organizational Leadership and Health Care Employee Burnout

and Satisfaction," *Mayo Clinic Proceedings* 95, no. 4 (2020): 698–708, https://doi.org/10.1016/j.mayocp.2019.10.041.

4.   J. H. Feingold, L. Peccoralo, C. C. Chan et al., "Psychological Impact of the COVID-19 Pandemic on Frontline Health Care Workers During the Pandemic Surge in New York City," *Chronic Stress* 5 (February 1, 2021): 2470547020977891, https://doi.org/10.1177/2470547020977891.

5.   Deloitte Centre for Health Solutions, "At a Tipping Point? Workplace Mental Health and Wellbeing," March 2017, https://www2.deloitte .com/content/dam/Deloitte/uk/Documents/public-sector/deloitte-uk -workplace-mental-health-n-wellbeing.pdf.

6.   J. B. Sexton, K. C. Adair, J. Proul, et al., "Emotional Exhaustion Among US Health Care Workers Before and During the COVID-19 Pandemic, 2019–2021." *JAMA Network Open* 5, no. 9 (September 1, 2022): https: //doi.org/10.1001/jamanetworkopen.2022.32748.

7.   K. I. Pollak, S. C. Alexander, J. A. Tulsky, et al., "Physician Empathy and Listening: Associations with Patient Satisfaction and Autonomy," *Journal of the American Board of Family Medicine* 24, no. 6 (2011): 665– 672, https://doi.org/10.3122/jabfm.2011.06.110025.

8.   F. Derksen, J. Bensing, and A. Lagro-Janssen, "Effectiveness of Empathy in General Practice: A Systematic Review," *British Journal of General Practice* 63, no. 606 (January 2013): e76–e84.

9.   P. J. Moore, N. E. Adler, and P. A. Robertson, "Medical Malpractice: The Effect of Doctor-Patient Relations on Medical Patient Perceptions and Malpractice Intentions," *Western Journal of Medicine* 173, no. 4 (October 2000): 244–250, https://doi.org/10.1136/ewjm.173.4.244; PMID 11017984; PMCID: PMC1071103.

10. C. J. Norris, "The Negativity Bias, Revisited: Evidence from Neuroscience Measures and an Individual Differences Approach," *Social Neuroscience* 16, no. 1 (2021): 68–82, https://doi.org/10.1080/17470919.2019 .1696225.

11. S. Southwick, L. Wisneski, and P. Starck, "Rediscovering Meaning and Purpose: An Approach to Burnout in the Time of COVID-19 and Beyond," *American Journal of Medicine* 134, no. 9 (2021): 1065–1067, https://doi.org/10.1016/j.amjmed.2021.04.020.

12. H. J. Tak, F. A. Curlin, and J. D. Yoon, "Association of Intrinsic Motivat-

ing Factors and Markers of Physician Well-Being: A National Physician Survey," *Journal of General Internal Medicine* 32, no. 7 (2017): 739–746, https://doi.org/10.1007/s11606-017-3997-y.

13. A. Alimujiang, A. Wiensch, J. Boss, et al., "Association Between Life Purpose and Mortality Among US Adults Older Than 50 Years," *JAMA Network Open* 2, no. 5 (May 3, 2019): e194270, https://doi.org/10.1001/jamanetworkopen.2019.4270.

14. T. D. Shanafelt, S. Boone, L. Tan, et al., "Burnout and Satisfaction with Work-Life Balance Among U.S. Physicians Relative to the General U.S. Population," *Archives of Internal Medicine* 172, no. 18 (2012): 1377–1385.

15. J. B. Sexton and K. C. Adair, "Forty-five Good Things: A Prospective Pilot Study of the Three Good Things Well-Being Intervention in the USA for Healthcare Worker Emotional Exhaustion, Depression, Work-Life Balance and Happiness," *BMJ Open* 9, no. 3 (March 1, 2019): e022695.

CONCLUSION

1. D. A. Mata, M. A. Ramos, N. Bansal, et al., "Prevalence of Depression and Depressive Symptoms Among Resident Physicians: A Systematic Review and Meta-analysis," *JAMA* 314, no. 22 (2015): 2373–2383, https://doi.org/10.1001/jama.2015.15845.

About the Author

PSYCHIATRIST JESSI GOLD, MD, MS, is the chief wellness officer of the University of Tennessee system and an associate professor in the department of psychiatry at the University of Tennessee Health Science Center. She is a fierce mental health advocate and highly sought-after expert in the media on everything from burnout to celebrity self-disclosure. Dr. Gold has written widely for the popular press, including for the *New York Times*, the *Atlantic*, *InStyle*, *Slate*, and *Self*. In her clinical practice, she sees healthcare workers, trainees, and young adults in college. A graduate of the University of Pennsylvania (with a degree in anthropology), the Yale School of Medicine, and the Stanford University department of psychiatry, she spends her free time traveling with her friends, watching live music or mindless television, and on walks with her dog, Winnie.

Find her on X, Instagram, Threads, and TikTok @drjessigold.